Rehabilitation

Commissioning Editor: Susan Young
Development Editor: Catherine Jackson
Project Manager: Andrew Palfreyman
Designer: Stewart Larking
Illustration Manager: Bruce Hogarth

Rehabilitation

The Use of Theories and Models in Practice

Sally Davis MSc RGN PGCEA DipMan

Programme Lead, Rehabilitation, School of Health and Social Care, Oxford Brookes University, Oxford, UK

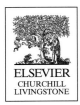

ELSEVIER
CHURCHILL
LIVINGSTONE

EDINBURGH LONDON NEW YORK OXFORD PHILADELPHIA ST LOUIS SYDNEY TORONTO 2006

ELSEVIER
CHURCHILL
LIVINGSTONE

First published 2006

ISBN 0 443 10024 1

British Library Cataloguing in Publication Data
A catalogue record for this book is available from the British Library

Library of Congress Cataloging in Publication Data
A catalog record for this book is available from the Library of Congress

Notice
Knowledge and best practice in this field are constantly changing. As new research and experience broaden our knowledge, changes in practice, treatment and drug therapy may become necessary or appropriate. Readers are advised to check the most current information provided (i) on procedures featured or (ii) by the manufacturer of each product to be administered, to verify the recommended dose or formula, the method and duration of administration, and contraindications. It is the responsibility of the practitioner, relying on their own experience and knowledge of the patient, to make diagnoses, to determine dosages and the best treatment for each individual patient, and to take all appropriate safety precautions. To the fullest extent of the law, neither the publisher nor the editor assumes any liability for any injury and/or damage.

The Publisher

Contents

Contributors

Sally Davis MSc RGN PGCEA DipMan
Programme Lead in Rehabilitation, School of Health and Social Care, Oxford Brookes University, Oxford, UK

Sally Feaver DipCOT BA MA
Principal Lecturer in Occupational Therapy, School of Health and Social Care, Oxford Brookes University, Oxford, UK

Mary Gottwald MA BA(Hons) TDipCOT CertEd(FE & HE)
Programme Lead Management in Health and Social Care, School of Health and Social Care, Oxford Brookes University, Oxford, UK

Michael K. Iwama PhD MSc BSc OT
Associate Professor, Department of Occupational Therapy, University of Toronto, Toronto, Canada; Adjunct Professor, University of Queensland, Australia

Mary Kavanagh MSc PGDip BA(Hons) DipCOT CertCounselling CertTHE
Senior Lecturer in Occupational Therapy, School of Health and Social Care, Oxford Brookes University, Oxford, UK

Sue Madden PhD BSc(Hons) SRP
Senior Lecturer in Physiotherapy, School of Health and Social Care, Oxford Brookes University, Oxford, UK

Kevin Reel MSc BSc PGDip CertTHE
Senior Lecturer in Occupational Therapy, School of Health and Social Care, Oxford Brookes University, Oxford, UK

Bridget Taylor MSc BA(Hons) RGN DNCert CertEd
Senior Lecturer in Sexual Health and Adult Nursing, School of Health and Social Care, Oxford Brookes University, Oxford, UK

Introduction

INTRODUCTION

Rehabilitation is a complex process which depends on interprofessional working and should be focused on the individual's goals (Sinclair and Dickinson 1998, Wade 1990, Steiner et al 2002). In order to achieve this there are a number of theories and models which can be used to make sense of rehabilitation and which can assist rehabilitation professionals.

It became obvious to me as a rehabilitation nurse and lecturer of a rehabilitation programme that a book exploring different models and their implications for rehabilitation could be useful for practitioners and educators. Hence the development of this book which aims to:

- Explore the use of theories and models in rehabilitation
- Identify the use of models in practice
- Facilitate interprofessional working
- Enable an approach that is focused on the individual.

Key features of this book are interprofessional working and how each model promotes this, and the ICF (International Classification of Function and Health, WHO 2001) which will be used to compare a variety of models against. The rationale for using the ICF is that it is a useful framework to use in rehabilitation as it considers a number of aspects related to the individual's experience.

The book is divided into three main sections: Rehabilitation; Models and Theories; Models in Practice.

Throughout the book four case studies are used to relate the discussion to practice. These case studies are taken from practice and are meant to cover different client groups, culture, ages and gender.

The authors of this book are from a variety of professional groups and have worked with a variety of client groups. The models chosen for the book are by no means an exhaustive list and the aim of this book is not to state that these models should be used in rehabilitation, it is to show how different models can be used to promote interprofessional working in rehabilitation. The rationale for choosing the models has come from the author's experiences in using models and also in wanting to explore the use of different types of models in rehabilitation.

Section One: Rehabilitation

Rehabilitation: Rehabilitation at a macro and micro level; definitions of rehabilitation; major government agendas; interdisciplinary and multidisciplinary teamwork; quality of life.

The ICF: The history; revisions; description; results of a survey; applications; relationship to rehabilitation.

Section Two: Models and Theories

Use of models: Terminology; use of theories; uni-professional models

Section Three: Models in Practice

This section will consider the following models focusing on how they promote interprofessional working; their relationship with the ICF; their relationship to rehabilitation.

The Canadian Model: A comprehensive, holistic model.

The Illness Constellation Model: Focuses on one aspect of rehabilitation: adaptation for the individual and their significant others.

The PLISSIT and Ex-PLISSIT models: Intervention models which help rehabilitation professionals in areas of sensitivity.

Health Promotion Models: Emphasising the link of health promotion to rehabilitation.

The Kawa (River) Model: Focusing on the cultural context of individuals.

This section will conclude with a focus on the Way Forward which will pull the main points of the book together, identifying areas for future development and research and the implications for interprofessional training.

It is anticipated that this book will be of value to:

- Professionals working in rehabilitation settings
- Professionals taking post-registration programmes in rehabilitation or programmes where rehabilitation is addressed e.g. ageing studies
- Students on pre-registration training for nursing and allied health professions
- Professionals working in any health care setting where interprofessional working is a focus.

In terms of terminology different chapters may use different terminology to describe the person undergoing the rehabilitation process. Generally client or individual is used rather than patient. I prefer the use of 'individual' as I feel patient and client implies different things. However, using 'individual' may be confusing at times which is why in some chapters client or patient is used.

Although there are limitations to this book in that it doesn't include an overview of all models available or includes all uni-professional models, hopefully it still has value in that it:

- Provides an overview of a variety of models with a focus on rehabilitation and interprofessional working
- Is multi-professional
- The ICF is used as a framework to compare the models against
- Is related to practice through the use of case studies and questions for practice
- Is in an accessible style.

I and my fellow authors hope that you enjoy the book and find it useful in considering the models you use in your practice. We also hope that it will challenge your thinking around the use of models in promoting interprofessional working.

Sally Davis

References

Sinclair A, Dickinson E 1998 Effective practice in rehabilitation: evidence from systematic reviews. Kings Fund, London

Steiner WA , Ryser L, Huber E, et al 2002 Use of the ICF model as a clinical problem-solving tool in physical therapy and rehabilitation medicine. Physical Therapy 82(11):1098–1107

Wade DT 1990 Designing district disability services – the Oxford experience. Clinical Rehabilitation 4:147–158

World Health Organisation 2001 International classification of functioning, disability and health. World Health Organisation, Geneva

SECTION **1**

Rehabilitation and the ICF

Chapter 1

Rehabilitation at a Macro and Micro Level

Sally Davis, Sue Madden

INTRODUCTION

Rehabilitation is a complex process that involves a number of health-care professionals, the individual and their family. Rehabilitation is becoming more of a priority in England with the formulation of National Service Frameworks, which prioritise rehabilitation in health care. The aim of this chapter is to set the scene for the book by discussing rehabilitation at a macro and micro level by:

- Discussing the history of rehabilitation
- Identifying the major government agendas related to rehabilitation
- Discussing what rehabilitation is both in terms of a process and a philosophy
- Exploring the related concepts of teamwork and quality of life.

REHABILITATION WITHIN THE CONTEXT OF SOCIAL POLICY

History of rehabilitation in the NHS

Rehabilitation is seen widely by many as being an essential part of a patient's care, as it is here that a person has the opportunity to fulfil his or her potential. However, prior to the launch of the NHS Plan in 2000, rehabilitation attracted little attention and was rarely mentioned within health and social policy, and, as a result, rehabilitation services received poor funding. The reduced funding was reflected in a reduction of rehabilitation services that resulted in a wide gap between the care provided within a hospital setting and that received once discharged back home and within the community. Because of the under-resourcing of rehabilitation, few areas had adequate services, which meant that individuals were unable to receive the support required.

Such underfunding and general lack of focus received by rehabilitation within health and social policy can be attributed to several issues. Traditionally, when clinical specialties needed rehabilitation services, whether these were clinical, therapeutic, social or environmental interventions, money would be allocated from each specific clinical specialty's budget to fund part of the service that was required. This traditionally resulted in one rehabilitation team providing a service to a number of clinical groups and specialties. While in theory this was a workable practice, because of structural issues the rehabilitation service was frequently unable to develop and progress as other clinical services could. Frequently, rehabilitation services lacked ownership, as one service could be funded by several clinical areas and, while the managers of each clinical specialty were often regarded as the managers of the service, this tended to be an implicit arrangement rather than being explicit. As a result, services became fragmented and lacked a clear sense of identity.

A further problem with such funding structure and lack of ownership was that frequently rehabilitation services were not regarded as a priority. As a result, when clinical services were making decisions about how to spend their budgets, it was frequently rehabilitation services that would be reduced, while other areas relating to acute services and long-term care were prioritised. Although this decision was viewed as necessary at the time, the underfunding of rehabilitation services had serious consequences within both the acute and long-term services, as patients had more frequent or longer stays in hospital, entry into residential care and nursing homes or needed more expensive and complex packages of support at home. One problem that emerged was that patients were receiving less rehabilitation while being treated as inpatients, as advances within clinical areas meant patients were spending less and less time as inpatients. As few rehabilitative services were provided within the community, upon discharge from the acute setting many people entered a downward spiral of being less independent and requiring more support. As funding became more problematic, particularly within the community setting, local authorities prioritised the small amount of funding on those most dependent and hence seen as most needing care. Not only were such packages of care more complex and more expensive but those who required lower levels of support were neglected, which led to those initially identified as being in need of little support deteriorating and becoming more likely to require expensive packages of care later on.

Because of such issues, the Audit Commission has repeatedly referred to rehabilitation as the Cinderella service of the NHS. While clearly being acknowledged as an essential service, the lack of ownership, funding issues and general perception that it is a low-priority service has led to its severe neglect. However, since the launch of the NHS Plan and subsequent National Service Frameworks such problems are being addressed. There is now widespread acknowledgement that the previous funding structures added to the stress placed on the NHS and social services, as limited resources were being used to fund expensive complex packages of care for people who had not had an adequate opportunity to achieve their full potential.

Increased recognition for the need of rehabilitation services

Since the launch of the NHS Plan in 2000, rehabilitation has become a priority within NHS policy, not least with the development of the National Service Framework for Older People and the establishment of intermediate-care services. The vision of the NHS set out within the NHS Plan is to provide a person-centred NHS that supports and enables people to live in an environment suitable to their needs that provides appropriate care, support and, if necessary, rehabilitation. The NHS Plan outlined that one of the key aims of a patient centred NHS should be to promote independence at all times. To achieve such independence, authorities, which includes social care authorities, should help individual adults to perform activities of daily living independently for as long as possible, and to live in their own homes for as long as possible. The NHS Plan identified that the only way such aims can be fully achieved is through rehabilitation services, which must include effective assessment of an individual's needs, on-going review and follow-up of care packages over a long period of time.

In the NHS Plan and the subsequent health and social care policies that have emerged from it, there has been widespread acknowledgement that, with the right rehabilitative services, acute NHS Trusts would benefit, as the number of acute admissions would decrease while ensuring earlier discharge was also possible if additional rehabilitation could be provided within the individual's community setting. Those individuals who lived in long-term residential or nursing home care were also considered as having great potential and being able to regain their independence if the appropriate rehabilitative services were provided. However, how and where such rehabilitation services should be provided could be seen as a complicated issue. To avoid confusion, the NHS Plan identified several key areas where rehabilitation services should be provided; these included more care provided within the community, particularly in the area of improving rehabilitation following discharge from hospital, providing more specialist intensive inpatient rehabilitation for people following strokes or major surgery and ensuring appropriate funding for intermediate care.

National Service Framework for Older People

Intermediate care

Of all the health and social care policies that have been developed by the Department of Health, the National Service Framework for Older People can be seen to have had one of the most dramatic influences on the rehabilitation agenda. It has helped to ensure that rehabilitation becomes a priority across health and social care. One of the key initiatives that helped to achieve this and that emerged from the National Service Framework for Older People was in the area of intermediate care.

Intermediate care was developed to try to cover a number of areas within the care of older people, although the primary aim was to maximise independent living for older people. However, intermediate care also saw the potential to promote faster recovery time from illnesses, prevent admission or readmission to acute NHS Trusts and reduce, wherever possible, the use of long-term care. Ultimately intermediate care was seen as a way of ensuring that people who would otherwise face a prolonged and unnecessary stay in hospital or an inappropriate admission to acute inpatient care, long-term residential care or continuing NHS in-patient care got an effective package of care that would promote independence for as long as possible. While all would support such aims, they are nevertheless ambitious. As a result, the government acknowledged that the primary way in which these could be realistically achieved was through timely and appropriate rehabilitation. Individuals need to receive a comprehensive assessment that would feed into a comprehensive care plan. The aim of any treatment should be to maximise independence and wherever possible to allow individuals to live at home.

In order to achieve such aims, rehabilitation services need to change in the way they are funded and developed if they are to be effective. As a result, intermediate-care services need to be developed in partnership between primary and secondary health care, local government services, in particular social care, and the independent sector, and should include a wide range of services in order to meet the needs of all users. Intermediate-care services require a range of appropriate professionals from health and social care to be involved from the start of the assessment process and to work within a single assessment framework, single records system and shared protocols. In order to promote such integrated care across a wide variety of agencies, the 1999 Health Bill changed the way in which budgets could be managed, and allowed budgets from NHS bodies and local authorities to be pooled, usually within primary care trusts, so that comprehensive and integrated rehabilitative services could be commissioned from one budget. Although budgets can be transferred, one agency now has overall control of the budget and commissioning process. This ensures that intermediate-care services have a clear identity and ownership, something that was problematic in the past and led to a decline in rehabilitative services. Integrated care also allows either health or social care to purchase both services if required, as previously such services were funded separately. All such changes have been designed to ensure that intermediate-care services, including rehabilitation, are patient-centred.

The potential for intermediate-care services is vast, which has led to the role and profile of rehabilitation within the NHS increasing. Because of the emphasis placed upon intermediate care in the National Service Framework for Older People and the role of rehabilitation within the Framework, it is now hoped that rehabilitation will remain on the agenda for health and social care services and that the previous problems that led to the neglect of rehabilitation are things of the past.

Whole-systems working: multidisciplinary and interdisciplinary working

As previously highlighted, in order for the aims of intermediate care to be achieved, the way in which health- and social-care professionals work together needed to be reviewed. Previous research had discovered that rehabilitation services that adopted a more unidisciplinary approach to care and lacked a cohesive team approach appeared to have many problems. Different information was shared with patients, frequently leading to a confused picture of what the problems and treatment approach was to be. There was a general lack of communication between different health- and social-care professionals and a general lack of agreement about the primary aims of rehabilitation. As a result, the services' effectiveness was limited. Because of such problems, it was felt that the only way to achieve a truly patient-centred approach, as highlighted within the NHS Plan, was to ensure that health- and social-care professionals worked more effectively within a team and to adopt an integrated approach to care.

Under the old funding structure, such an integrated care approach was difficult to achieve, as professionals were funded from different budgets; hence establishing and building effective teams was almost impossible to achieve. However, within the new funding structure established within intermediate care it was now possible to bring all key health- and social-care professionals to work as a team, ensuring that the service was truly client-centred.

A further advantage with working within an integrated team approach to care is that the combined expertise of the team can be more effectively used than when health and social care workers practise individually. Each rehabilitation service should review the skills of all staff involved, such as medical, nursing, therapy and pharmacy staff, to ensure all professionals are used appropriately and that potential overlap of roles is reduced. A further shift in working patterns within intermediate care is that, to ensure that the service is truly client-centred, there will naturally be some blending and blurring of the roles adopted by health-care professionals. Although individual professional groups will remain distinct from one another, such flexibility will ensure that the needs of the individual are readily met.

However, the new integrated approach to care goes further than simply the rehabilitation team working within a particular service. There is also a need to ensure that all agencies involved with an individual's care work in an integrated approach, which means bringing together health and social care as well as other agencies, such as housing. One of the problems when different agencies work in isolation is that they frequently hold different views of the purpose of rehabilitation and have different aims. For example, while social services and education staff play a vital role in assisting people with rehabilitation needs to become integrated into society, they may hold a view of rehabilitation that is different from that of many health professionals working within the NHS. As a result, all agencies must come together to ensure an integrated approach to care. Only then can the whole care system be appropriately analysed, identifying possible areas for improvement, which in turn will make more acute and long-term beds available and ultimately reduce the cost of long-term care. Only by adopting such a truly integrated approach to rehabilitation can the needs of the individual be truly met and the services be delivered in a seamless manner.

REHABILITATION

There are many definitions of rehabilitation within the literature (Jackson 1984, Waters 1986, Wade 1990, Greenwood et al. 1993, Blackwell 1994, Sinclair & Dickinson 1998) but they all highlight similar defining attributes of rehabilitation:

Process

Rehabilitation is generally described as being an active, dynamic, continuing process concerned with physical, social and psychological aspects. Steiner et al (2002) characterise rehabilitation as a continuous process and identify the 'rehab cycle', which aims to improve an individual's health status and quality of life by minimising the consequences of disease. The cycle consists of five stages:

- Identifying problems and needs
- Relating the problems to factors that are limiting and can be modified
- Defining target problems and target mediators and selecting appropriate measures
- Planning, implementing and coordinating interventions
- Assessing effects.

The last stage of the cycle may cause new problems and needs to be identified, in which case the cycle begins again.

Restoration

In relation to rehabilitation, 'restoration' involves enabling the individual to regain lost elements of their life, such as physical functioning or personal and social identity. It also carries the sense of restoring the individual to society or to a purposeful and satisfying life. The use of the word 'restore' can imply that the emphasis of rehabilitation is on the individual returning to their former life. However, the definitions tend to interpret 'restore' in terms of individuals adapting to changed circumstances and learning new skills rather than returning to their former life roles. Pryor (2002) identifies rehabilitation as being the reconstruction of individuals' lives in the light of injury, illness or surgery. She sees rehabilitation as being about lives that are lived in damaged or broken bodies.

Effectiveness

Rehabilitation is described as promoting effectiveness or optimal functioning for the individual. Optimal functioning is implied as being functioning that can be achieved given any limitations the individual may have. Functioning could be interpreted in terms of emotional and psychological functioning as well as physical functioning.

Enabling and facilitating

Rehabilitation is generally described as being an enabling and facilitating process rather than a 'passive, doing for' process. This is conducive to rehabilitation being active rather than passive. In order for healthcare professionals to take on this enabling and facilitating role the relationship between them and the individual may need to be different. An interesting question is: where does the power lie in this kind of relationship?

Learning and teaching

Learning and teaching is implied within some definitions, in terms of rehabilitation being described as an educational process that enables patients and carers to learn new skills. Wade (1990) describes it as an educational, problem-solving process aimed at reducing disability and handicap. This is using the old International Classification of Impairments, Disability and Handicap (ICIDH; World Health Organization 1980) terminology. Applying the International Classification of Functioning, Disability and Health (ICF; World Health Organization 2001), this could be interpreted as increasing an individual's activity and participation.

Autonomy

Autonomy is implied in some of the definitions, in terms of enabling individuals to achieve goals that are important to them. However it is only the Kings Fund definition (Sinclair & Dickinson 1998) that stresses that rehabilitation should be a process aimed at restoring personal autonomy in those aspects of daily living considered most relevant by individuals and their family carers. This idea of restoring personal autonomy fits in well with goal planning and the concepts of empowerment and advocacy. Taking autonomy one step further, Cardol et al (2002) suggest that autonomy should be the ultimate aim of rehabilitation. In order for this to happen, health-care professionals will need to explore the concepts associated with autonomy – e.g. power, empowerment – and their implications.

The International Classification of Functioning, Disability and Health

Rehabilitation can be considered in terms of the ICF (World Health Organization 2001) under the classifications of impairment, activity and participation. Rehabilitation goals will be different related to each level. Using the ICF as a framework for rehabilitation ensures that the focus of rehabilitation is not only on the level of impairment and disability. It needs to focus on the individual's participation in the environment and in society. The goals at each level of the ICF will generally relate to each other. For example for an individual who has had a stroke the goals at each level might be as listed in Table 1.1.

The goals identified at the level of participation may be dependent on the achievement of goals at the levels of impairment and activity. The ICF in relation to rehabilitation is discussed in more detail in Chapter 2.

Table 1.1 Relationship of ICF categories to goals

ICF Category	Goal
Impairment	To regain function in hemiplegic arm and to prevent complications
Activity	To be independent in washing and dressing
Participation	To be able to return to work

Philosophy

As well as a process, rehabilitation can also be considered as being a philosophy of care. It is about the way professionals think about individuals and where they see their role in the process. As a philosophy, rehabilitation is about enabling, facilitating, empowering. Adopting this philosophy of rehabilitation means that health-care professionals:

- Value the patient as an individual, identifying their strengths and weaknesses; their past achievements; their hopes for their future. This is vital if professionals are to deliver client-centred care. Using assessment tools that assess individual's strengths, weaknesses, etc. can help to promote this value.
- Adopt strategies that facilitate and enable the individual to achieve their full potential. It is important that there is some continuity in the strategies used by rehabilitation professionals and that there is agreement as to what constitutes facilitating and enabling strategies.
- Realise that, although it may be necessary to devote more time to enabling individuals to achieve their full potential, this will be cost-effective in the long term. It can be difficult to take this view, particularly in an environment where rehabilitation is not seen as a priority. The time involved is perhaps the most common factor identified by health-care professionals in acute settings as a barrier to rehabilitation. However, health-care professionals need to consider whether this is a valid argument when set against the consequences of not promoting rehabilitation, both for the individual and for health-care resources. Not promoting rehabilitation in the acute setting may mean, for example, that the individual will not achieve their full potential given their limitations and will therefore need more resources and support after being discharged.
- Should be thinking about how the individual and their family will manage in the future, even though the extent to which they are able to affect the individual's level of participation may be limited. The focus should be on individuals' future quality of life as they see it.

Stages of rehabilitation

One of the remaining difficulties is that rehabilitation can be seen as something that happens in a specialised unit or ward whereas in reality it needs to commence the moment an individual enters the health-care system. This may be at the first contact with the GP or as an emergency case in Accident & Emergency. It can be helpful to consider this continuum of rehabilitation as having four stages. The aims of rehabilitation are different at each stage.

Stage 1

This is the initial critical stage when the individual is unconscious. The goal of rehabilitation at this stage is to preserve life. Interventions at this stage include:

- Preventing complications
- Providing verbal and tactile stimulation
- Supporting relatives.

Stage 2

At this stage the individual has recovered consciousness, is fully responsive and is beginning to regain some physical function. The goal of rehabilitation depends on the individual's needs. It may be to maintain a safe, comfortable environment, which may be an appropriate goal for an individual with a head injury who is agitated, or it may relate to the individual's functional and cognitive ability. Interventions may include:

- Managing challenging behaviour
- Assessing the individual's functional and cognitive ability
- Establishing everyday activities, e.g. eating at a table, using the toilet rather than a commode
- Giving the individual choices, e.g. about diet, clothes
- Establishing alternative forms of communication
- Supporting and involving relatives.

Stage 3   A more active programme of rehabilitation is required at this stage, which may take place in a rehabilitation ward or centre. The goals of rehabilitation should be focused on the level of participation – being concerned with the individual's quality of life. This will involve:

- Facilitating and enabling individuals to achieve their maximum potential in washing, dressing, feeding, communication and mobility
- Ensuring that there is continuity of therapy programmes between the different professional groups within the team
- Empowering individuals by giving them informed choice and by involving them in the setting of rehabilitation goals
- Providing psychological support to the individual and their family
- Providing a supportive, structured environment for the individual and family.

Stage 4   The individual will have reached their full potential at this stage. The focus will now be on enabling them to live with the disabilities they have and maintaining their quality of life in relation to work, hobbies and social life. At this stage they will either be at home or in an alternative setting, e.g. a nursing home. They may attend a young disabled unit for respite care or other day facilities, where the role of the team is to help them maintain their quality of life. In order for individuals to maintain their full potential, they may need follow-up appointments with the rehabilitation team, which may result in further assessments and interventions.

Rehabilitation and disability   Looking at rehabilitation in terms of four stages highlights the need for rehabilitation to be a team activity. The goals of rehabilitation at each stage will depend on the individual's impairments and the resulting disability or the limitations that the impairment places on their activities. Because of the effect the individual's disabilities can have on the rehabilitation process and outcomes it is useful to consider the relationship between rehabilitation and disability. Baker et al (1997) facilitated a survey of education needs of health and social-services professionals that explored the views of professional and client groups on the meaning of rehabilitation and disability. As a result of the survey disability was identified as being a dramatic life change for the individual, with rehabilitation being an enabling process in which a range of groups in society worked to meet the needs of the disabled person. This life change includes the way in which individuals see themselves and others. The report emphasised that disability should be related to the individual person with a disability rather than 'the disabled'. The use of language is an important consideration. The term 'the disabled' is still used in the media and in literature. This kind of language can be seen as discriminatory, as it implies that disabled people are not seen as individuals but are defined by their disability.

There are views in the literature on the relevance of rehabilitation to people who are disabled. Some of these views highlight the inadequacies of the World Health Organization (1980) ICIDH framework, which did not take into account the societal factors that disable individuals. The ICF (World Health Organization 2001) has rectified this by including the idea of level of participation, which identifies environment and societal factors. This enables disabilities to be described from the perspective of an individual's life circumstances and the impact these have on their experience (Bornman 2004). The focus on environmental and social factors fits in with Pryor's (2002) description of the creation of a 'rehabilitative milieu', by which she means an environment that enhances the process and outcome of rehabilitation. To enable this environment to be created, thought has to be given to the participants, the activities and the setting in which they take place (Pryor 2002).

It is interesting to consider whether definitions of rehabilitation reflect the cultures of different countries. For example, in some countries rehabilitation may be seen as synonymous with physiotherapy. In my experience, some professionals and individuals in the UK also hold this view. The goal of promoting autonomy and independence may not be congruent with the beliefs of individuals from different cultures. For example, a study undertaken by Stopes-Roe & Cochrane (1989, cited in Holland & Hogg 2001) comparing Asian people's attitudes to family values with those of white people in the UK found that Asian people valued conformity and self-direction less than the people in the UK. This may not be congruent with the concepts of autonomy and independence. It is therefore essential that rehabilitation is focused on the individual's needs and goals and that their values and beliefs are taken into account. It cannot be assumed that all individuals or professionals have the same views about rehabilitation. In order for professionals to deliver culturally competent rehabilitation care (Patrinos & White 2001) they need to:

- Be aware of their own attitudes towards diversity and examine these attitudes
- Be sensitive to and respect differences
- Be knowledgeable about different cultures to enable them to interpret behaviours appropriately
- Have cultural skills that enable them to respect and value culture – this may include the use of appropriate touch and non-touch when communicating and respecting the individual's need for physical space
- Be able to communicate cross-culturally, which may mean the involvement of interpreters or people in the community.

Focusing on what is important to the individual and what their goals are transcends all cultures.

TEAMWORK

Rehabilitation, because of its complex nature, cannot be achieved by one professional group alone. Rehabilitation has become synonymous with teamwork. A review of the literature on trends in rehabilitation policy (Nocon & Baldwin 1998) highlighted the need for rehabilitation to be centred on the most important aspects of an individual's life with the involvement of service users. To enable this to be achieved rehabilitation needs to involve a group of professionals all working with the same purpose of meeting the individual's goals. This process must involve the individual and their family. The Kings Fund definition of rehabilitation: 'a process aiming to restore personal autonomy in those aspects of daily living considered most relevant by patients or service users, and their family carers' (Sinclair & Dickinson (1998, p.1)) also highlights the need for a multiprofessional approach to rehabilitation. This definition also focuses on individual-centred care, emphasising what service users and their carers, not the professionals, see as important.

The five main principles of individual-centred care can be identified as being empowerment of individuals, enhancement of staff, multidisciplinary integrated pathways, multidisciplinary teamwork and restructuring and decentralisation of services (Hutchings et al 2003). One could argue that truly individual-centred care requires interdisciplinary teamwork in which there is not only a shared philosophy and collaboration but also blurring of professional roles in order to meet the individual's goals. This use of terminology brings into question the different terms used when talking about rehabilitation. Terms such as multiprofessional, interprofessional, transprofessional, multidisciplinary, interdisciplinary and transdisciplinary are often used interchangeably. What is the difference between professional and disciplinary? Between multi- and inter-? Table 1.2 gives some dictionary definitions.

'Multi-' implies that there are a number of different professional groups working together, whereas 'inter-' implies that there are a number

Table 1.2   Definitions of team types

Term	Definitions of Team Types (*Oxford Paperback Dictionary* 1998)
Professional	Someone who belongs to a profession, which is an occupation that involves knowledge and trainig at an advanced level of learning
Disciplinary	Of or for a discipline, which is described as training that produces a particular skill; or a branch of learning or instruction
Multi-	Involving many
Inter-	Between or among

of different professionals working together towards a common purpose and that there is some blurring of boundaries. 'Professional' can be taken to mean the different professional groups whereas 'disciplinary' can be taken to refer to the knowledge and skills underlying different professional roles. This is supported by Payne (2000), who distinguishes between 'professional' and 'disciplinary' by suggesting that 'professional' is concerned with the functions and activities associated with the different professional groups, whereas 'disciplinary' is concerned with the knowledge and skills required for different professional roles.

Norrefalk (2003) takes on the challenge of trying to make sense of the different terminology and identifies that:

- A multidisciplinary team
  - Involves the efforts of individuals from a number of disciplines
  - Is used to describe a team consisting of many different professions working in rehabilitation
- In an interdisciplinary team
  - Members not only require the skills of their own disciplines but also have the added responsibility of the group effort on behalf of the activity or individual involved
  - The skills necessary for group interaction are required, and the knowledge of how to transfer integrated group activities into a result that is greater than the simple sum of the activities of each individual discipline
  - The group activity is synergistic
- In a transdisciplinary team
  - All borders are broken between the individual professionals. One member of the team acts as a primary therapist, being supported by the rest of the team. This primary therapist may be a health-care assistant with specific rehabilitation training (Jackson & Davies 1995).

The terms 'discipline' and 'professional' can be identified as having more or less the same meaning. Norrefalk (2003) makes the point that it is important that rehabilitation professionals nationally and internationally use the same terminology with the same meaning. He makes the suggestion that 'multiprofessional team' is used rather than 'multidisciplinary team'. As the team consists of different professionals, this does perhaps make sense. However, there can still be seen to be a difference between 'multi-' and 'inter-', with the interprofessional team truly working across boundaries in order to meet the goals that are important to the individual and have been identified by them. This fits in with the view of McGrath & Davis (1992), who consider the distinction between multidisciplinary and interdisciplinary to be their focus, with 'multidisciplinary' being focused on the level of activity and 'interdisciplinary' focused on the level of participation. It is the level of participation that enables goals to be more realistic for the individual. In rehabilitation, professionals should be working towards goals that are important to the individual.

Collaboration

Collaboration is the key to effective team working and can be described as the process of working towards a common goal with shared planning and action. The team has joint responsibility for the outcome (Lindeke & Block 1998). Interdisciplinary collaborative care differs from multidisciplinary collaborative care in that it involves joint decision making, shared responsibility and shared authority (Lindeke & Block 1998). Professionals work together and cooperatively to achieve an agreed individual-centred goal. Transdisciplinary care takes this way of working one step further in that there is a complete blurring of goals with one person being responsible for ensuring that the individual's needs are met (Hutchings et al 2003). Although collaboration is the ultimate aim in practice it is not always easy to achieve. Freeman et al (2000), as a result of looking at case studies of six teams, identified that difficulties in developing collaborative practice can be identified at the levels of the organisation, the group and the individual. There are a number of concepts that affect all these levels, which need to be taken into account for collaboration to occur. Figure 1.1 identifies concepts related to collaboration, which are the basis for a taught module on collaboration at the School of Health and Social Care, Oxford Brookes University.

Although team working is seen as being central to rehabilitation there is little published evidence for its effectiveness (Embling 1995, Waters & Luker 1996, Proctor-Childs et al 1998). There is evidence at a clinical level from professionals who have changed from one approach to another that it does have an effect on individuals (McGrath & Davis 1992). Using a case study approach, Proctor-Childs et al (1998) explored the realities of multi- and interdisciplinary teamwork. Although this was a small study using only two case studies, both from a neurorehabilitation setting, the findings support the work of McGrath & Davis (1992). Proctor-Childs

Figure 1.1   Concepts related to collaboration

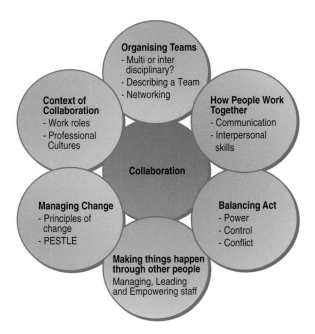

et al (1998) identified the following six outcomes that have the potential to enhance an individual's progress:

- *Continuity*: Professionals learned skills and knowledge from each other, which they then carried over into their own practice
- *Consistency*: Achieved because professionals identified how other team members interpreted events – this resulted in them being able to 'pick up' on individuals' views and act in a similar way to colleagues
- *Reduction of ambiguity*: The same messages were given to individuals and their families because of joint working, joint discussion and joint evaluation
- *Appropriate referrals*: Professionals had a greater knowledge of each other's roles so were able to refer appropriately to other members of the team
- *Holistic information*: A holistic picture of the individual was achieved because of joint working – because of the perspectives of a number of team members, decisions were made from a wider knowledge base
- *Problem solving*: As discussion was focused around specific aspects of individual care joint strategies were developed and appropriate decisions made.

In order to achieve the above outcomes the team needs to be a close working team, comfortable with each other, motivated by the same philosophy. Using the social identity approach to team building identified by Hayes (2002) could help achieve this. This approach has three main aims:

- To motivate the team by creating a sense of unity and belonging. This then enables them to cooperate together to achieve team goals, which would need to be aimed at patients' goals

Strategies: Ensure the team is well defined and that there is cooperation with others in the organisation; define the team's resources clearly; set mutually agreed boundaries for the team
- To create a climate of mutual understanding to enable team members to be aware of each other's contribution and to see how individual skills, abilities and tasks contribute to the team as a whole

Strategies: Establish clear lines of communication and different strategies for communication; be clear what the team's aims and objectives are; identify opportunities for informal communication, e.g. social activities
- To enable team members to feel proud of belonging to their team and to recognise their contribution to the organisation

Strategies: Appraise each other's successes to each other and to the larger organisation; recognise each other's skills and abilities; provide training opportunities for individuals and for the whole team; have official recognition from the wider organisation, which could be in the form of rewards.

The implications of this approach to teams is that team building must be a priority and must address:

- *Attitudes, values and beliefs*: Team members exploring these in relation to rehabilitation and to team working
- *Trust and respect*: Setting ground rules within teams
- *Role*: Team members having the opportunity to explore their understanding of each other's roles
- *Contributions*: Team members need to see how their contribution affects not only the team but also the wider strategic picture.

Using such an approach to team building could help rehabilitation teams truly achieve interdisciplinary working.

QUALITY OF LIFE

The ultimate aim of rehabilitation can be identified as maximising an individual's quality of life. That is, the quality of life that is important to the individual, not what professionals think it should be. Quality of life is a difficult concept to define as it is personal to the individual. What is important to one person will not have the same importance for another person. In conducting a concept of analysis of quality of life, Meeburg (1993) concluded that quality of life is an overall satisfaction with life as determined by the individual whose quality of life is being evaluated. Meeburg (1993) gives the example of a person living in poverty who may be happy with their life as they have known nothing else. However, a person outside those conditions would evaluate that person's life as less than ideal. This example, however, doesn't take into account people whose quality of life has changed as a result of circumstances beyond their control, e.g. illness, trauma, bereavement, financial difficulties.

To understand the complexity of the concept of quality of life it is helpful to consider its attributes or characteristics as identified by the concept analysis conducted by McDaniel & Bach (1994).

- *Dynamic nature*: Quality of life may change at various stages or ages in an individual's life. It may also change from day to day. This is important to consider in terms of rehabilitation, as an individual's quality of life may be affected by a number of factors including the rehabilitation process itself, lack of resources and the process of adaptation. These effects may be short- or long-term.
- *Multiple dimensions*: Quality of life is made up of a number of dimensions, for example physical functioning, social interaction, family and friends. The importance these dimensions have for individuals will be different. This means that it is vital that the team identifies what is important to the individual and what they see as a priority in terms of the different dimensions of their quality of life.
- *Interaction*: The interaction between the individual and their environment may influence their quality of life. Environment can be thought of as the rehabilitation environment, the home environment and the community environment. Attitudes can also be considered as part of the environment.

● *Congruence*: Quality of life is affected by the difference between an individual's hopes and expectations and their actual life. This can be a major influence on the quality of life of people with chronic illness and/or a disability, and is a factor that needs to be considered by rehabilitation professionals.

These characteristics identify quality of life as more than an overall satisfaction with life. McDaniel & Bach's (1994) content analysis identified quality of life as a dynamic, unique process that is influenced by the dimensions of an individual's life. It is the product of the congruence or lack of congruence between the individual's hopes and expectations and their actual life conditions. It is interesting to consider whether different populations see quality of life in a different way. Lau et al (2003), in a study defining quality of life for elderly Chinese people who had had a stroke, identified that there were similarities and differences in the qualify of life components identified in the study. The study identified 36 components, which can be classified using the ICF categories (Table 1.3). Some components can be listed under more than one category.

To obtain these components the following questions were asked in the study:

● What does it mean for you to have a good life?
● What are your reasons for saying so?
● Apart from [what was said], what other aspects do you feel are important for you to have a good life?
● How would you rate your own life? What are your reasons for saying that your life is [very poor, poor, fair, good, very good/excellent]? (Lau et al 2003, p. 711)

Table 1.3 ICF categories and components of quality of life

Body Function and Structures	Activities and Participation	Environmental Factors	Personal Factors
Limb function	Activity participation	Working capacity	Happiness
Bowel and bladder function	Activities of daily living	Formal social support Social integration	Dependence on medication/treatment
Vision and hearing Language ability	Dependence on medication/treatment	Physical safety and security	Self-concept: body image
Cognition	Personal relationships	Housing	Self-concept: self-worth
Pain and discomfort	Sexuality	Finance	
Energy and fatigue	Informal social support	Transport	Coping
Sleep and rest		Physical environment	Spirituality
	Opportunities for new information and skills	Leisure	Life satisfaction Sense of control
	Sense of acceptance		Negative feelings

Source: With permission from Lau et al 2003

To assess what quality of life means for individuals, health-care professionals could use these questions more generally. In terms of the differences in quality of life for Chinese and Western populations, Lau et al (2003) identified that the main differences were in the areas of 'eating/appetite', 'being accepted/respected' and 'family', which Lau et al (2003) felt were due to sociocultural factors.

Identifying quality of life as incongruence between the hopes and expectations of individuals and their actual life conditions highlights the need for rehabilitation health-care professionals to work with individuals to narrow the gap between what they want and what is actually possible.

One way of doing this is to consider quality of life as being made up of the roles we as individuals have in life. It is these roles that make up our quality of life. Role theory can be used to explain the roles individuals assume during various situations (Chin 1998). It is these roles that govern an individual's behaviour in a group and determine their relationships with other group members. The roles that individuals have can be categorised as primary, secondary and tertiary (see Fig. 1.2).

Focusing on what is most relevant to the individual means that rehabilitation has to be concerned with that individual's quality of life. It is necessary for the team to establish what is required to enable individuals to return to their former roles in life or to establish new ones in order to achieve an acceptable quality of life. One way of doing this is to enable the identification of life goals. In a literature review of 39 articles on life goals and their influence on the rehabilitation process, Sivaraman Nair (2003) concluded that:

- Individuals strive either to attain or to avoid life goals
- The participation in the rehabilitation programme maybe influenced by life goals
- It is not clear whether rehabilitation outcomes are improved by the focus on life goals.

Although there is a need for further studies into the effect of life goals on the rehabilitation process, life goals is one way of ensuring that the

Figure 1.2   Categorisation of roles

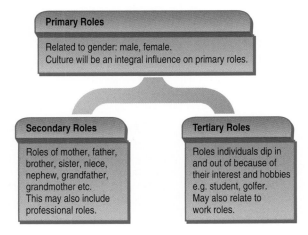

Primary Roles

Related to gender: male, female.
Culture will be an integral influence on primary roles.

Secondary Roles

Roles of mother, father, brother, sister, niece, nephew, grandfather, grandmother etc.
This may also include professional roles.

Tertiary Roles

Roles individuals dip in and out of because of their interest and hobbies e.g. student, golfer.
May also relate to work roles.

rehabilitation programme is focused on what is important to the individual and their quality of life.

One concept to consider in terms of control is autonomy, which implies a sense of control and can be seen as central to quality of life. However, the choices they have and the resources available can limit autonomy for individuals. This may highlight ethical issues, for example the ethics of rehabilitation professionals enabling and encouraging individuals to take control and be autonomous when the resources required for them to do so, in terms of facilities, equipment and financial support, are not available. It may then be that professionals are setting individuals up to fail. A way of avoiding this is for rehabilitation professionals and individuals to negotiate control and support, which would then acknowledge the disempowered state of both individuals and rehabilitation providers (Clapton & Kendall 2002).

Wellness is an interesting concept to consider in relation to quality of life. Wellness can be identified as a dynamic process that integrates physical and psychosocial development, spirituality and the environment (Drayton Hargrove & Derstine 2001). Wellness can be achieved without physical independence. Perhaps quality of life is about achieving a level of wellness that is appropriate for the individual and that is identified by the individual. Putnam et al (2003) conducted a study to explore how people living with long-term disabilities defined health and wellness. The 99 adults in the study had a variety of disabilities including polio, cerebral palsy, multiple sclerosis, amputation and spinal cord injury. Focus groups were used to explore health promotion practices, barriers and opportunities to being healthy and well. The participants defined health and wellness as being independent or self-determining; being able to do what they wanted to do; having an emotional and physical state of well being; and being free from pain. The results highlighted the fact that the state of being healthy and well is not solely dependent on the individual but is associated with the cultural, social and physical environment.

CONCLUSION

With the introduction of the NHS plan and the National Service Frameworks, the amount of rehabilitation work being carried out within the National Health Service has increased, the focus being on an integrated approach involving rehabilitation and social services.

Rehabilitation is a complex process, which needs to actively involve the individual, their family and the team and commence at the acute stage. The focus of rehabilitation needs to be on health, wellness and quality of life. In terms of quality of life, rehabilitation needs to focus on goals that are important to the individual. However, the concepts of autonomy and control need to be taken into account. It is also important that health-care professionals consider rehabilitation as a philosophy of care as well as a process.

Teamwork is essential to rehabilitation; the team must work collaboratively with the individual towards the individual's goals. It is essential that rehabilitation professionals value and take into account the needs of individuals and understand their beliefs and values. More research is needed into the effectiveness of interdisciplinary and multidisciplinary teamwork on rehabilitation.

QUESTIONS FOR DISCUSSION

- How do you ensure that rehabilitation is focused on the individual's quality of life?
- As a team, how do you see rehabilitation? Is it a process? A philosophy? When does it begin?
- How do others in your hospital or Trust see rehabilitation? Is there a consistency in their views?
- Do any aspects of the social identity approach apply to you as a team?

References

Baker M, Fardell J, Jones B 1997 Disability and rehabilitation: survey of education needs of health and social services professionals. Disability and Open Learning Project, London

Blackwell 1994 Blackwell's dictionary of nursing. Blackwell Scientific Publications, Oxford

Bornman J 2004 The world health organisation's terminology and classification: application to severe disability. Disability and Rehabilitation 26:182–188

Cardol M, DeJong BA, Ward CD 2002 On autonomy and participation in rehabilitation. Disability and Rehabilitation 24:970–974

Chin PA 1998 Theoretical bases for rehabilitation. In: Chin PA, Finocchiaro D, Rosebrough A (eds) Rehabilitation nursing practice. McGraw-Hill, New York

Clapton J, Kendall E 2002 Autonomy and participation in rehabilitation: time for a new paradigm? Disability and Rehabilitation 24:987–991

Department of Health 1999 Health Bill. HMSO, Norwich

Department of Health 2000 The NHS Plan: a plan for investment, a plan for reform. HMSO, Norwich

Department of Health 2001 National Service Framework for Older People. HMSO, Norwich

Drayton Hargrove S, Derstine JB 2001 Definition and philosophy of rehabilitation nursing: history and scope including chronicity and disability. In:

Derstine JB, Drayton Hargrove S (eds) Comprehensive rehabilitation nursing. WB Saunders, Philadelphia

Embling S 1995 Exploring multidisciplinary teamwork. British Journal of Therapy and Rehabilitation 2:142–144

Freeman M, Miller C, Ross N 2000 The impact of individual philosophies of teamwork on multi-professional practice and the implications for education. Journal of Interprofessional Care 14: 237–247

Greenwood R, Barnes MP, McMillan TM et al 1993 Neurological rehabilitation. Churchill Livingstone, Edinburgh

Hayes N 2002 Managing teams: a strategy for success. Thomson Learning, Southbank, Victoria

Holland K, Hogg C 2001 Cultural awareness in nursing and health care. Edward Arnold, London

Hutchings S, Hall J, Lovelady B 2003 Teamwork: a guide to successful collaboration to health and social care. Speechmark, Bicester

Jackson HF, Davies M 1995 A transdisciplinary approach to brain injury rehabilitation. British Journal of Therapy and Rehabilitation 2:65–70

Jackson MF 1984 Geriatric rehabilitation on an acute care medical unit. Journal of Advanced Nursing 9:441–448

Lau ALD, McKenna K, Chan CCH et al 2003 Defining quality of life for Chinese elderly stroke survivors. Disability and Rehabilitation 25:699–711

Lindeke LL, Block DE 1998 Maintaining professional integrity in the midst of interdisciplinary collaboration. Nursing Outlook 46: 213–217

McDaniel RW, Bach CA 1994 Quality of life: a concept analysis. Rehabilitation Nursing Research Spring:18–22.

McGrath J, Davis A 1992 Rehabilitation: where are we going and how do we get there? Clinical Rehabilitation 6:225–235

Meeburg GA 1993 Quality of life: a concept analysis. Journal of Advanced Rehabilitation 18:32–38

Nocon A, Baldwin S 1998 Trends in rehabilitation policy: a review of the literature. King's Fund, London

Norrefalk J 2003 How do we define multidisciplinary rehabilitation? Journal of Rehabilitation Medicine 35:100–101

Oxford Paperback Dictionary 1998 The Oxford paperback dictionary, 3rd edn. Oxford University Press, Oxford

Patrinos DS, White N 2001 Culturally competent rehabilitation care. In: Derstine JB, Drayton Hargrove S (eds) Comprehensive rehabilitation nursing. WB Saunders, Philadelphia

Payne M 2000 Teamwork in multiprofessional care. Palgrave, Basingstoke

Proctor-Childs T, Freeman M, Miller C 1998 Visions of teamwork: the realities of an interdisciplinary approach. British Journal of Therapy and Rehabilitation 5:616–618, 635

Pryor J 2000 Creating a rehabilitative milieu. Rehabilitation Nursing 25: 141–144

Putnam M, Geenen S, Powers L, et al 2003 Health and wellness: people with disabilities discuss barriers and facilitators to well being. Journal of Rehabilitation 69: 37–45

Sinclair A, Dickinson E 1998 Effective practice in rehabilitation: evidence from systematic reviews. Kings Fund, London

Sivaraman Nair KP 2003 Life goals: the concept and its relevance to rehabilitation. Clinical Rehabilitation 17:192–202.

Steiner WA, Ryser L, Huber E et al 2002 Use of the ICF model as a clinical problem-solving tool in physical therapy and rehabilitation medicine. Physical Therapy 82: 1098–1107

Stopes-Roe M, Cochrane R 1989 Traditionalism in the family: a comparison between Asian and British cultures and between generations. Journal of Comparative Family Studies 20:141–158

Wade DT 1990 Designing district disability services – the Oxford experience. Clinical Rehabilitation 4:147–158

Waters KR 1986 The role of the nurse in rehabilitation. Care-Science and Practice 5:17–21

Waters KR, Luker KA Staff perspectives on the role of the nurse in rehabilitation wards for elderly people. Journal of Clinical Nursing 5:103–114

World Health Organization 1980 International classification of impairments, disabilities and handicaps. World Health Organization , New York

World Health Organization 2001 International classification of functioning, disability and health. World Health Organization, Geneva

Chapter **2**

The International Classification of Function and Health

Sally Davis, Sue Madden

INTRODUCTION

The World Health Organization (WHO) devised the International Classifi-cation of Functioning and Health (ICF) in 2001 as a reclassification of the International Classification of Impairments, Disabilities and Handicaps (ICIDH). The ICF is being used in rehabilitation centres to structure the rehabilitation process. The aim of this chapter is to:

- Explore the history of the ICF, its revisions and the rationale behind them
- Describe the classification and the theories that underpin it
- Explore the uses of the ICF
- Explore its relationship to rehabilitation – this will include the results of a survey of rehabilitation professionals.
- Relate the ICF to four different case studies.

THE INTERNATIONAL CLASSIFICATION OF IMPAIRMENT, DISABILITY AND HANDICAP

Although the ICF has only recently emerged from the WHO (World Health Organization 2001), it has in fact emerged from several alterna-tive classifications, which can be traced back to the 1980s. The earliest classification system from the WHO was the ICIDH, which was pub-lished in 1980 and is widely accepted to be the first system that attempted to define and classify the impact chronic illness has upon an individual's body. One of the main purposes of the ICIDH was to offer an alternative classification system to the then well established Interna-tional Classification for Diseases (ICD). The aim of the ICD was, and still remains, to classify illnesses in terms of diagnoses and pathological abnormalities and, while it remains a well accepted and useful tool used by health-care professionals dealing with people with acute illnesses, conditions that were more chronic in nature appeared, under the ICD classification system, to have less relevance. As a result, the ICIDH was developed to help standardise the way in which the impact of chronic illness upon an individual was classified. When first published, the ICIDH was considered to be a useful tool across rehabilitation, medicine and social welfare, primarily because it was the first classification system that attempted to deal with the complex issues relating to the consequences of illness. The ICIDH has become key to UK policy and, since its initial publication in 1980, has been used across a range of health-care initiatives, including health outcomes research, population surveys, coding health information and vocational assessment and as an organisational basis for social policy.

Impairment, disability and handicap

In order to classify the impact chronic illness has upon an individual, the ICIDH presented three levels of classification:

Disease/disorder $\rightarrow$ impairment $\rightarrow$ disability $\rightarrow$ handicap
    ICD   ICIDH   ICIDH   ICIDH

Impairment, as the first classification within the ICIDH, was concerned primarily with abnormalities of body structure, appearance and organ or system function. As a result, impairment was defined as an abnormality or disturbance of any cause that occurred within the body, which is then subsequently experienced by the body. Hence impairment was seen and defined at the level of the body. The second level of classification, disability, is seen as a consequence of impairment and is considered in terms of functional performance and activity by the individual. Hence, disability is seen not to be at the level of the body, as is the case with impairment, but is regarded as being at the level of the person. The final level of classification is handicap. Handicap is classified according to the impact the impairment and disability has upon the individual in terms of the person's relationship with their environment. It was therefore argued that handicap was concerned with and measured how a person with a disability was able to interact and adapt to their surrounding environment. Impairment as a classification was used as the basis of the ICIDH, which was divided into nine chapters that focused upon the following impairments: intellectual; psychological; language; aural; ocular; visceral; skeletal; disfiguring; generalised; sensory and other impairments. This reinforced the notion that disability and handicap occurred as a consequence of an impairment.

The terms, definitions and relationships of impairment, disability and handicap were developed by the authors of the ICIDH as it was their belief that these were more applicable to individuals with chronic illness, and clinicians involved in their treatment, than the classification system of diagnosis represented by the ICD. It was therefore argued that the ICIDH was established to classify the illness not simply in terms of a diagnosis but by the way in which the condition impacted upon an individual's body. Nevertheless, as impairment was seen to emerge as a result of disease/disorder within the body and the subsequent relationship between diagnosis, impairment, disability and handicap, when the ICIDH was initially presented it was done so to support the classification of the ICD and was encouraged to be used with it. It was then down to individual clinicians whether to use the ICD or the ICIDH, a decision that should be influenced by their area of work.

When the ICIDH was published, it was anticipated that it would be used for a number of purposes. Among the functions of the ICIDH were to help to identify the long-term impact that disease has upon individuals, to identify the frequency at which particular health-care services are used for certain conditions, and to help to organise medical notes on the basis of the classifications used. A further function, and one that was central to its development, was that, by standardising the way in which chronic illnesses were classified, it would make it possible to evaluate the effectiveness of health care within chronic conditions. It was also anticipated that, by providing a universally accepted model that classified the impact of disease upon an individual, the authors and the WHO hoped that the terminology and definitions of concepts would be standardised, thereby making it more possible to compare data collected across countries.

Limitations of the ICIDH

As might be anticipated, creating an internationally accepted classification for the impact of chronic illness is, by its nature, problematic. Although when the ICIDH was initially published in 1980 the authors invited and anticipated criticism, the amount received was vast, which ultimately led to revisions and the ICF, which was published in 2001. In order to understand the subsequent revisions and the emergence of the ICF, it is important to consider why such revisions were necessary.

One of the major criticisms surrounding the ICIDH was the way in which impairment, disability and handicap were defined. According to the authors of the ICIDH, one of the original aims was to challenge the medical model by moving the focus away from the diagnosis and pathological condition within a person's body and to look at the consequences of that condition upon the body. The ICIDH wanted disability and handicap to be more of a focus within the health-care agenda and to have more attention paid to how such conditions were impacting upon people, particularly in terms of the effect disability can have upon social exclusion. In this sense, the authors argued that the ICIDH was the opposite of the medical model. However, critics of the ICIDH have argued the contrary. The fact that impairment, disability and handicap are all determined by a disease or disorder within an individual's body clearly links the ICIDH with the medical model, with many arguing that its very foundations are in the medical model. As with the medical model, the ICIDH and ICD function on the basis that clearly defined norms exist; those outside such predefined norms are classified as having a disorder, impairment, disability or handicap, or, as social commentators would define it, as having some type of deviant behaviour away from normal society.

A further argument supporting the notion that the ICIDH is an extension of the medical model is the definition of impairment, disability and handicap. The definitions appear to emphasise the individual's role within their disability, in the sense that, if the impairment impacts upon what a person is able to achieve, then they are defined as having a disability. As a result, it is the individual who determines whether they are disabled or not, with little attention paid as to how the environment may impact upon the person's level of disability. Although the definition of impairment attempts to address the role of the environment within the disability, the emphasis remains with the individual, as it is defined by how the individual interacts with and adapts to their environment. Because of the focus placed upon the individual, the ICIDH appears to support the notion that it is the individual's responsibility to adjust to the disability and to find appropriate coping strategies that allow them to function within their environment. A problem then emerges when trying to use the ICIDH as evaluating the effectiveness of health-care interventions. Because social environments are not fully acknowledged within the level of disability, and are limited within the level of impairment, it is difficult to state whether a change that may occur in a disability and handicap classification is due to the rehabilitation received from health-care workers or to changes in the social environment of the individuals with the disability. As a result, a key function of the ICIDH appears to be undermined.

A further problem within the ICIDH was that it was developed with no input from the disability movement group. One of the biggest criticisms of the classification from disability groups and others independent of these is that the language used within the classification is negative, particularly the term 'handicap'. A further problem with the ICIDH from the perspective of the disability movement groups was the lack of acknowledgement of the social model of disability within the classification. Frequently, disability movement groups argue, disability is a socially constructed phenomenon imposed on people by society in which the biggest challenge comes from their environment, both physically and mentally, and not from the individual's illness. If the environment was more accessible in a physical and mental sense, then a person would immediately be less disabled and handicapped. Regardless of how well a person may be able to cope with their impairment, the environment immediately limits a person's ability to function within society as they may wish to.

Although most would suggest that the medical model and social model of disability have a role to play within the construction of disability, the fact that the ICIDH was developed from the view of the medical profession led to it being universally rejected by disability movement groups. With such a large group rejecting the ICIDH, the long-term future of the model was bought into serious question, which was in part why revisions were made.

Revisions of the ICIDH

In 1992, it was agreed that the ICIDH needed to be revised in the light of the criticisms that had been made. When the ICIDH was republished in 1993, the WHO agreed that the original version had not paid sufficient attention to the role of the environment and that this need to be revised. There was also some confusion as to the exact relationship between impairment, disability and handicap, which also needed to be revised. A further argument as to why the revision was appropriate arose from developments in health care in terms of treatment and rehabilitation and the wide range of people who were accessing such health-care provision. As the number of people with long-term conditions increased, the need for a classification that incorporated the diversity of users needed to be revisited. The WHO also argued that revisions were needed because the ICIDH was being used in ways for which it had not been designed; therefore, as the function of the ICIDH was expanding, these should be incorporated within a new version.

Between spring 1996 and spring 1999, three new versions of the ICIDH were produced. The alpha version was followed by beta-1 in 1997 and beta-2 in 1999; these are collectively referred to as ICIDH-2. All the revised versions aimed to provide a common language to describe functional states associated with frequently encountered health conditions. The ICIDH-2 also aimed, by using neutral terminology, to improve communications between health-care workers, other sectors and people with disabilities. It was also hoped that the ICIDH-2 would promote better care and services that would focus on improving the participation in society of people with disabilities.

Despite the revisions, a number of disability organisations in North America continued to cite several key arguments against the ICIDH and ICIDH-2. One of the continued arguments was the fact that disability was defined in medical terms, whereby a disabled person is viewed as not normal. In a sense, a person must enter into the sick role, access medical health-care services and follow health-care workers' advice. Although the sick role may allow an individual to be excluded from social obligation, the sick person also has to give up social rights and, once they have entered the health-care world and are defined as being ill, they will always remain so. However, many people with disabilities argue that they are healthy and have no cause to access medical services. Disability movement groups also remained concerned that a health-care worker could define a person in terms of a disability and by doing so had a degree of control over their life, particularly in terms of social rights, while also making judgements on the quality of life an individual might or might not enjoy.

Despite such criticism from the disability movement groups, the authors of the ICIDH-2 do acknowledge that, while many people with a disability lead healthy lives and medical intervention would have no influence over the quality of those lives, it would also be a mistake to ignore the effect that appropriate medical interventions can have on other people's quality of life. Indeed, the authors argue that the most urgently required care modalities for people with disabilities are medical and rehabilitation care.

THE INTERNATIONAL CLASSIFICATION OF FUNCTIONING, DISABILITY AND HEALTH

The ICF can be described as a component of health classification, rather than a classification of the consequences of disease, as the ICIDH was. It is intended to be universal, concerning all people irrespective of health condition and age. The aim of the ICF is to classify health and health-related states by using categories within health and health related domains. The ICF describes the situation of each person with different health-related domains within the context of environmental and personal factors. It systematically groups health and health-related domains. It provides a systematic coding scheme to code different health and health-related states and permits the comparison of data between health-care professionals and across countries. The WHO recommends that users have training in how to use the classification.

The ICF consists of two parts covering functioning and disability and contextual factors. Within each part there are two components, which can be expressed in positive and negative terms. These components also consist of various domains and constructs.

Human functioning in the ICF is identified as operating at three levels:
- Level 1: at the level of the body or body part
- Level 2: the whole person
- Level 3: the whole person in a social context.

Disability exists when there is dysfunctioning at one or more of these levels.

Functioning is the umbrella term used to cover positive aspects of the ICF, i.e. body functions, structures, activities and participation, whereas disability is used to cover the negative aspects – impairments, activity and participation limitations. Disability is identified as being the result of impaired interaction between individuals and the environment (Bornman 2004).

The two parts of the ICF are Part 1: Functioning and Disability and Part 2: Contextual Factors (Table 2.1). In the classification, each component of the ICF has different chapters covering different aspects of the component. These chapters have codes allocated to them.

Table 2.1   Overview of the ICF

	Part 1: Functioning and Disability		Part 2: Contextual Factors	
Components	Body function and structures	Activities and participation	Environmental factors	Personal factors
Domains	Body functions and structures	Life areas (tasks, actions)	External influences of functioning and disability	Internal influences on functioning and disability
Constructs	Change in body functions (physiological)	**Capacity:** executing tasks in a standard environment **Performance:** Executing tasks in the current environment	Facilitating or hindering impact of features of the physical, social and attitudinal world	Impact of attributes of the person
Positive aspect	Functional and structural integrity Functioning	Activities Participation	Facilitators	Not applicable
Negative aspect	Impairment Disability	Activity limitation Participation restriction		

Body functions, structures and impairments

- Body functions: the physiological and psychological functions of body systems and structures
- Body structures: organs, limbs and their components: anatomical parts of the body
- Impairments: problems in body structure or function, e.g. weakness in left arm, paralysis of lower limbs. Impairments can be temporary or permanent; intermittent or continuous; progressive, regressive or static. Impairments may result in other impairments; for example, movement functions may be impaired by lack of muscle power. If an individual has an impairment it doesn't necessarily mean that they have a disease or are sick.

Chapter titles: body functions

1. Mental functions
2. Sensory functions and pain
3. Voice and speech functions
4. Functions of the cardiovascular, haematological, immunological and respiratory systems
5. Functions of the digestive, metabolic and endocrine systems
6. Genitourinary and reproductive functions
7. Neuromusculoskeletal and movement-related functions
8. Functions of the skin and related structures

Chapter titles: body structures

9. Structure of the nervous system
10. The eye, ear and related structures
11. Structures involved in voice and speech
12. Structure of the cardiovascular, immunological and respiratory systems
13. Structures related to the digestive, metabolic and endocrine systems
14. Structure related to genitourinary and reproductive systems
15. Structure related to movement
16. Skin and related structures

Activities and participation, limitations and restrictions

- Activities: the execution of an action or task by an individual, e.g. preparing a meal, getting dressed
- Participation: the involvement of the individual in a life situation, e.g. going shopping, socialising with friends
- Activity limitations: the difficulties an individual may have in performing activities, e.g. unable to wash, dress
- Participation restrictions: the difficulties an individual may experience in life situations, e.g. socialising, at work.

A single list covers a range of life areas for activities and participation. Qualifiers are used in terms of performance and capacity to distinguish between what an individual can do in their environment and what their ability is in executing a task or an action.

Chapter titles: activity and participation

1. Learning and applying knowledge
2. General tasks and demands
3. Communication

4. Mobility
5. Self-care
6. Domestic life
7. Interpersonal interactions and relationships
8. Major life areas
9. Community, social and civic life.

Contextual factors

Environmental factors make up the environment in which people live and conduct their lives in terms of physical, social and attitudinal environment, e.g. social attitudes to disability, physical access to buildings and services, integration into the community, opportunities for socialising. In the classification, environmental factors are focused on two levels:

- Individual: referring to the immediate environment of the individual, e.g. work, school, home – this includes contact with others, e.g. family, peers, strangers
- Societal: the formal and informal social structures, services and systems that impact on the individual in the community or society – this includes government agencies, transportation services and regulations.

Body functions interact with environmental factors, e.g. interactions between air quality and breathing, sounds and hearing.

Chapter titles: environmental factors

1. Products and technology
2. Natural environment and human-made changes to environment
3. Support and relationships: people or animals that provide practical, physical or emotional support
4. Attitudes: external to the individual, not their own attitudes. Attitudes observable as a result of customs, practices, ideologies, values, norms, religious beliefs
5. Services, systems and policies: public, private, voluntary services at community, regional, national or international level.

Personal factors

Personal factors are the internal factors that have an impact on how an individual is experiencing disability, e.g. gender, age, coping styles, social background, education, profession, past and current experience. This is the particular background of an individual, how they live their life. It will consist of features that are not part of a health condition. Personal factors are not classified in the ICF. No rationale is really given for this except for difficulty of classifying them.

Disability and functioning are viewed as outcomes of interactions between health conditions and contextual factors, which include environmental and personal factors. This is a shift in thinking away from the medical model to the social model. The WHO describes the model the ICF is based on as a biopsychosocial model, which is an integration of the medical and social model. This acknowledges that disability is complex, involving the body and the environment. For some individuals, disability will be entirely internal, while for others it will be external. This view of the need for both the medical and social model is supported by

Goodall (1995) in her suggestion of an interface model which accepts the individual variations of a framework to underpin the Universal Declaration on the Human Genome and Human Rights (1997), which is that everyone has a right to respect for their dignity and a right to be respected for their uniqueness and diversity. The social model is not a new idea; it has been around for many years being championed by people who are disabled as an alternative view to the medical model. Although perhaps it has taken some time, the ICF does recognise the effects of the social model. As Hurst (2003) says, it also provides a framework that can be developed.

Figure 2.1 represents the model of disability that the ICF is based on. It reflects the interactions between the health condition and the ICF concepts. As can be seen, most of the interactions are two-way: for example, an individual's health condition can affect their body functions and structures, their activities and their participation. These may also in turn affect their health condition. Also, body functions and structure, activities and participation may affect environmental and personal factors and at the same time environmental and personal factors can affect an individual's activities and participation.

THEORIES RELATED TO THE ICF

It is not explicit what if any theories underpin the ICF. But it is useful to consider the main theories used to underpin conceptual models and see how they fit in with the ICF.

Systems theory   A system can be identified as components that interact with each other within any particular period of time (Buckley 1967, cited in Hymovich & Hagopian 1992). The individual can be identified as a system consisting of systems (e.g. circulatory, respiratory), interacting with other systems (e.g. family, environment). The ICF identifies systems in terms of

Figure 2.1   Body functions, structures and impairments Source: Reproduced from World Health Organization 2001 with permission of the World Health Organization; all rights reserved by the Organization.

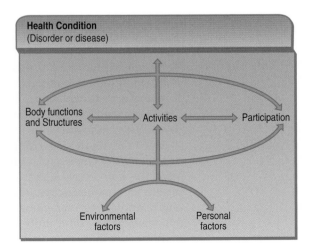

body structures, environmental and personal factors. Perhaps an intervention by health-care professionals might be to look at how these systems are interacting with each other and how this can be managed. For example, if an individual is blind a change in their body structure may affect how they interact with the environment. Existing models emphasising this theory are the Contingency Model of Long-Term Care (Hymovich & Hagopian 1992), King's Open System Model (King 1981), Neuman's Systems Model (Neuman 1982) and the Model of Human Occupation (Kielhofner 2002).

Adaptation theory

Adaptation theories view change as being the interaction between the person and the environment in terms of cause and effect. Adaptation theory helps us to understand what causes balance in the equilibrium and what the effects are of a disturbed equilibrium (Leddy & Pepper 1989). Roy's adaptation model (Roy 1984) identifies the set of processes that are used by an individual to adapt to environmental stressors. This model views the individual as being in constant interaction with a changing environment. Adaptation is the process individuals go through in dealing with a stressor. Individuals use different coping mechanisms to adapt to a stressor. How people cope is different for each individual and can be seen as being individual to them. This links in with the ICF in terms of personal factors. Factors such as age, gender, culture and lifestyle may affect the way a person adapts to a stressor. Coping styles is also mentioned in the ICF, as a personal factor that needs to be taken into account. The way an individual deals with stressors may have an effect on the outcome and on the intervention.

Motivational theory

One of the personal factors that can affect the rehabilitation process for an individual is motivation. Motivational theory (Maslow 1968, cited in Hoeman 1996) identifies that there are a number of factors that can influence an individual's motivation. Within the ICF motivation is identified in terms of mental functions that produce the incentive to act; the conscious or unconscious driving force for action. It is categorised under body functions. The ICF can help identify the factors that might affect an individual's motivation, e.g. the environment, physical independence and ability to participate in activities, personal factors.

Role theory

Roles can be identified as sets of expected behaviours or patterns (Chinn 1998). In different situations individuals will assume different roles. Role theory can help explain the interactions and roles individuals and their families assume when they are confronted with a stressor such as disability or illness.

The effect on the individual if they are unable to resume valued roles or if their roles change is an important element of rehabilitation and could affect the way people adapt. This links in with the ICF to a degree in terms of activities and participation, with the focus on interpersonal interactions and relationships, engagement in education, work and employment, and engagement in community and social life. However one of the areas identified by WHO for further development is quality of life.

Self-care theory

Self-care theory identifies self-care actions as being activities that individuals perform to maintain health and well being (Orem 1985). Individuals act in a manner that will maximise their health, by learning and performing activities that will support their health (Davis & O'Connor 2004). Personal self-care is essential for individuals to be able to develop a sense of self-worth and independence.

It is in Orem's model of nursing (Orem 1985) that the concept of self-care and self-care deficit theory has been developed and implemented by nurses. Orem not only identifies self-care in her theory but also talks about:

- Self-care deficits, where individuals are unable to perform self care due to limitation
- Self-care agency, which is the individual's ability to perform self-care and may be affected by factors such as motivation, age, skills and knowledge
- Therapeutic self-care demand, which includes the actions required by the individual to maintain health
- Other agencies – the ability of health-care professionals to provide the care required by the individual.

In relation to the ICF, the codes allocated to the constructs enable health-care professionals to assess an individual's level of self-care and also to monitor that self-care. In terms of self-care being affected by other factors, the ICF also enables health-care professionals to consider these factors in terms of the environment and personal factors.

USES OF THE ICF

The ICF is meant to cover the lifespan but has not been used extensively in studies involving children. Ogonowski et al (2004) looked at the inter-rater reliability in assigning ICF codes to children with disabilities in the USA. This was the first of a number of studies looking at how the ICF can be used effectively with children with disabilities. The study involved 60 children with a range of developmental disabilities ranging in age from 9 months to 17.75 years. Researchers rating the six domains in the Activities and Participation component considered 40 codes. Three paediatric functional assessment tools were used to assess the children and then it was determined which of the 40 codes applied to each child, on the basis of items from the assessment measures. The results of the study suggest that it is feasible to use existing functional assessment tools to apply some of the codes from the Activities and Participation components. However the researchers were unable to achieve a level of agreement on many of the codes. Ogonowski et al (2004) recommend the development of alternative functional assessment tools.

It seems to be at the level of activity and participation that current research is focusing. Parenboom & Chorus (2003), in a literature review, investigated which existing survey instruments assessed participation. They found nine instruments that measured participation to some extent, but only two involved most of the items at participation level.

They concluded that more discussion was needed to distinguish between activity and participation.

Jette et al (2003) conducted a survey of 150 adults aged 60 plus living in the community in the USA to identify distinct concepts within physical functioning that fit in with the activity and participation levels. Physical functioning assessment instruments were used to collect data. Jette et al (2003), along with Ogonowski et al (2004) and Parenboom and Chorus (2003), highlight the need for further development of the ICF and development of assessment tools that measure the specific constructs within the ICF.

A study describing the use of the ICIDH and the subsequent ICF by nursing and allied health professionals in the Netherlands (Heerkens et al 2003) concluded that the ICF was too general to be used to describe the functioning of the individual at the level of detail needed by healthcare professionals. The authors cited as an example the fact that knowing that an individual has a problem 'washing the whole body' does not help the nurse or occupational therapist to know where the problem lies. Is it not being able to handle the soap, being unable to reach all parts of the body or not knowing the right order of actions involved?

In terms of intervention the ICF can be used to determine whether a particular intervention programme has been effective at the levels of body function and structure, activity and participation (Bornman 2004). The ICF can help to emphasise the strengths of individuals with a disability by focusing on their participation in a particular environment; it can assist individuals to participate more extensively through interventions aimed at enhancing their competence by removing barriers and increasing facilitators in the environment; it can provide an indication of the environmental and personal factors that might hamper participation (Bornman 2004).

Relationship to rehabilitation

Rehabilitation is a continuous process, which involves identifying problems and needs, and relating these problems to impaired body functions and structures, the factors of the person and the environment. The process also includes the management of rehabilitation interventions (Stucki et al 2002). If the aim of rehabilitation is to maximise an individual's quality of life to what they want, then rehabilitation needs to focus on more than impairment and disability. It has to take into account the environment and the context that individual comes from. The ICF gives rehabilitation professionals a framework to enable them to do this.

The focus on quality of life has to stem from the beginning of the rehabilitation process, which ideally should be during the acute stages. This can be achieved by identifying goals for participation, involving the family and taking into account contextual factors (Rentsch et al 2003). Although there are elements identified in the ICF that relate to quality of life, quality of life itself is not considered (Wade & Halligan 2003). Wade & Halligan (2003) suggest an expanded WHO ICF model of health and illness that includes a description of quality of life. The expanded model includes other concepts that have an effect on quality of life such as happiness and role satisfaction. Wade & Halligan (2003) identify the need for the construct of free will to be added as a capacity.

The ICF enables rehabilitation to move away from illness towards health, making it a more positive process. Because of its focus on health, the ICF can also enable rehabilitation professionals to adopt more of a health promotion focus. The model in Figure 2.2 highlights how health promotion and rehabilitation can work together. It is based on the results from a study undertaken with rehabilitation nurses on their understanding of health and health promotion (Davis 1995). It can help rehabilitation professionals identify the concepts more specifically.

Health promotion   Within the model health promotion and rehabilitation are concerned with promoting wellness no matter what the individual's limitations in activities and participation are. Wellness can be equated with wellbeing, which is described in the ICF as encompassing all those aspects that make up a 'good life'. This includes physical, social and mental aspects. Domains of wellbeing are identified as being education, employment, environment, etc.

In order to promote health promotion, rehabilitation professionals need to address the following issues:

Figure 2.2   Health promotion model for nurses working in neurological rehabilitation

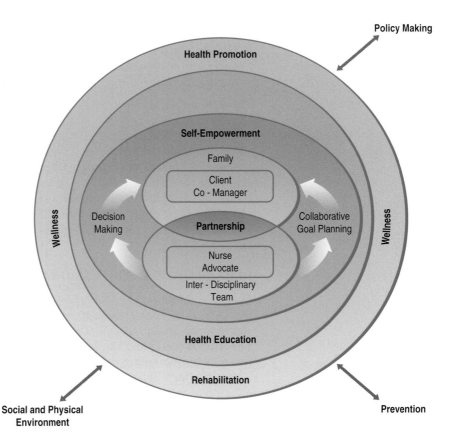

- Social and physical environment: access to leisure facilities; people with disabilities having the same access in the environment as people without disabilities; access to adequate support services and resources to enable individuals to return to their own environment; support groups in the community for individuals and their families; support for employers to enable individuals to return to work
- Prevention: active enforcement of seat belt and drink/driving laws; stronger penalties for drink driving; screening for high blood pressure; family planning advice; education on diet, alcohol, drugs, smoking and accident prevention
- Policy making: equal opportunities policies for people who are disabled; policies related to alcohol and tobacco advertising; policies related to new buildings.

These issues relate to the contextual factors in the ICF.

Health education

The aim of health education within health promotion is to empower individuals by providing them with information and decision-making skills. Health education activities include:

- Promotion of independence: self-care activities; mobility; collaborative goal planning; instructing the individual and their family
- Adaptation to lifestyle: counselling including sexual counselling; psychological support; teaching new skills; managing stress
- Health maintenance: nutrition, dental hygiene and physical exercise; avoidance of toxic substances, e.g. smoking, drugs and alcohol; management of epilepsy; monitoring blood pressure and blood glucose.

These issues relate more to the activity and participation factors in the ICF.

Individuals

Within the model individuals are identified as being co-managers of their rehabilitation programme with control over their own health. The amount of control may vary with other factors, e.g. the environment, other people's attitudes. This is in keeping with the contextual factors of the ICF. The family is recognised as being an important part of the individual's life if that is what the individual wants. The relationship between the individual and the team is one of partnership.

REHABILITATION PROFESSIONALS AND THE ICF

The rehabilitation professional's role is one of informing and supporting individuals to enable them to make decisions. This role involves interdisciplinary goal planning. The ICF can be used to ensure that individual-centred goal planning is a reality and that the team are focusing on more than functioning, taking into account contextual factors as well.

It is perhaps easier to see how the ICF framework will be adopted as a common language and will be used to guide assessments, goal planning, etc. than how the classification will be used, although the ICF does provide health-care professionals with a coding system that, although it could be seen as time consuming to use, with development could be used to guide assessment and interventions. Stucki et al (2002) make the point that the success of the ICF as an agreed global language will depend on its acceptance by rehabilitation practitioners. An unpublished survey conducted in 2001 at an international conference for rehabilitation nurses gives some insight into the usage of the ICIDH framework and practitioners' awareness of the ICF. Although mainly a nursing conference the participants consisted of other health-care professionals.

Results of survey

Unpublished survey, 2001: 108 questionnaires.

Five questions were asked, with space for comments. The results will be discussed under each question:

Question 1. What area of health-care practice do you work in and what country?

96 out of 108 participants responded to this question. The majority of participants were from the UK, with participants from England, Scotland and Wales. The main areas of people's work were neurological rehabilitation; stroke services and elderly rehabilitation. The questionnaire didn't ask for the respondent's professional group. It can be assumed that most of the respondents were nurses, with a small number of physiotherapists and occupational therapists (Table 2.2).

Table 2.2   Respondents' area of health-care practice and country

Area	Total no.	Country
Neurological rehabilitation	29	England: 20; Australia: 7; Scotland: 7; Ireland: 1
Stroke services	16	England: 12; Scotland: 4
Elderly rehabilitation	14	England: 7; Scotland: 5; Wales: 2
Rehabilitation medicine	7	England: 3; Wales: 4
Community rehabilitation	7	England: 6; Scotland: 1
Orthopaedic	4	England: 4
Lecturers	4	England: 3; Wales: 1 (learning disabilities)
Physical disability	3	England: 3
Private sector	3	England: 1; Scotland: 2
Day hospital	2	England: 1; Scotland: 1
Renal	1	England: 1
Back pain rehabilitation	1	England: 1
Amputee rehabilitation	1	England: 1
Multiple sclerosis	1	England: 1
Palliative care	1	England: 1
Rehabilitation administration	1	USA: 1
Not specified	1	Isle of Man: 1

Question 2. Do you use the ICIDH framework in your clinical area? If so how?

The answers were No = 94, Yes = 14. Of the 14 respondents who said they did use the ICIDH in their clinical practice, 12 identified specifically the following areas: Teaching (3), Audit(1), Planning patient goals (4), Identifying outcomes (2), Administration (1), Clinical practices (1).

Question 3. Are you aware of the revision of the ICIDH to the ICF?

91 respondents said No and 17 said Yes.

Question 4. Has this had any impact on your practice? If so how?

The answers were: No = 40, Yes = 8, Not applicable = 21, No answer = 39. Of the eight respondents who answered Yes, seven said that the revision had impacted on their practice in the following areas:

- Admission
- Auditing teams' records
- Outcomes' measurement and goal setting
- Policy development
- Teaching
- Physiotherapists using it
- Setting up rehabilitation services
- Changing practice.

Question 5. Do you think it could make a difference to your practice? If so how?

The responses were No = 4, Yes = 44, Unsure = 36, Not applicable = 1, No answer = 23. 23 respondents identified ways in which the framework could make a difference to their practice. These can be categorised as listed in Table 2.3.

Comments on the ICF

The following comments were made on the ICF:

- 'Keep it simple and user friendly'
- 'It looks similar to occupational therapy models'

Table 2.3 Areas where the ICF framework might make a difference to practice

Area	Possible Improvement
Assessment and outcomes	Assessment guidelines: outcome measurement
Audit	Evaluation of service; setting standards; guide to best practice
Common language: goal setting	To organise patient goals
Improving documentation	Enabling the team easier access to what is important for the patient re: quality of life; better dissemination of information to the team
Discharge	To pick up on social problems rather than focus on function
Staff levels	In terms of patient dependence
Service planning	Describing the needs of client groups
Shift focus of team to health and participation	Make the team less disease focused; clarify the disease process; giving patients more independence and self-esteem

- 'Needs training time'
- 'Looks like a lengthy process'
- 'As with all models, it is the way it is applied to practice that makes it workable'
- 'Fingers crossed it helps us really focus on what is important'.

Conclusions

Although this was a small survey and specialised, in that it targeted a certain group, some conclusions can be drawn from it that are useful to consider, particularly as the use of the ICF is currently under study.

It is interesting that only 13% of the conference delegates used the ICIDH in practice. One might have expected this percentage to be higher in light of the literature advocating the use of the ICIDH in rehabilitation (Post et al 1999, Gray & Hendershot 2000, Wade 2001, de Kleijn-de Vrankrijker 2003). Only 15.7% were aware of the revision of the ICIDH to the ICF, which maybe is not surprising as in 2001 the revision was only just being publicised. In terms of practice, 7.4% said that the ICF had had an impact on their practice in terms of admission, auditing, outcomes' measurement, goal setting, policy development and teaching. In terms of the difference it could make to practice, 40.7% thought it would make a difference. Interestingly 33.3% were unsure and 12% didn't answer. This could indicate the need for supply of information and knowledge about the ICF to health-care professionals to enable them to see how the ICF could be relevant to their practice.

The areas identified by the respondents where the ICF might make a difference equate with the views in the literature:

- Assessment and outcomes (Cieza et al 2002, Heerkens et al 2003)
- Audit (Stucki et al 2002, Kearney & Pryor 2003)
- Common language (Dahl 2002, Stucki et al 2002, de Kleijn-de Vrankrijker 2003, Rentsch et al 2003)
- Documentation (Heerkens et al 2003, Kearney & Pryor 2003, Rentsch et al 2003)
- Discharge (Rentsch et al 2003)
- Staffing levels
- Service planning (Crews & Campbell 2001, Dahl 2002, Stucki et al 2002, Hurst 2003)
- Shift of focus (Hurst 2003).

The conclusions that can be drawn from the survey are that the ICF could be very useful for rehabilitation, as it enables health-care professionals to focus on health and participation rather than on illness and disability and provides them with a common language. The ICF could enhance the rehabilitation process in terms of assessment, outcomes, discharge and service planning. However, the respondents did identify the need for the ICF to be user-friendly and for it to be a shorter process. The need for training to use the ICF relates to Bornman's (2004) view, which categorises the ICF as a complex coding system.

CASE STUDIES

The last section in this chapter will consider four case studies in relation to the ICF in an attempt to relate the preceding discussion to practice. These case studies will also be used throughout the book to demonstrate different models and issues.

CASE STUDY JOEY

Joey is a 50-year-old single unemployed man who lives with his partner on the tenth floor of an apartment block. His partner, John, works as a self-employed plumber. Joey has been unemployed for the last 18 months. He has always enjoyed cooking and now has decided to do all the cooking as it makes him feel that he is contributing to the partnership and therefore increases his self-esteem and makes him less anxious and stressed. However, during his period of unemployment he has put on 4 stone. Joey has recently recovered from a heart attack and is now back at home.

Changes in body functions and structures

There are changes in Joey's heart in terms of a weak valve. The main change in body function is that Joey is no longer able to undergo any major physical exertion, e.g. running for any length of time, climbing a large number of stairs.

Activities and participation

Capacity

- Before the heart attack Joey led generally a sedentary lifestyle, going out only to go to the shops. He had an active sexual relationship with John. Since the heart attack, Joey's capacity has only changed in terms of him not being able to climb stairs or run.

Performance

- Joey's actual performance since the heart attack is not much different from before his heart attack. His performance changed when he lost his job, in that he was not as active as he had been and was less motivated.
- Since the heart attack Joey has not been able to climb stairs and he and John have not resumed their sexual relationship.

Environmental factors

- Joey and John have always had to put up with the negative attitude of some of the tenants in the apartment block. Since Joey's heart attack this has worsened, with homophobic graffiti being written on the walls.
- Although there is a lift to the flat, this is occasionally not working, which in the past meant that Joey had to walk up ten flights of stairs. Following his heart attack Joey is afraid to leave the flat in case the lift isn't working when he gets back.

Personal factors

- Joey has lost motivation since he became unemployed. He has found comfort in eating, which has resulted in him putting on weight.
- Joey is generally an anxious person. He worries about what other people think of him. He is not secure in his relationship with John. This has worsened since he became unemployed and had the heart attack. He feels that John doesn't find him attractive and will look elsewhere.

CASE STUDY CHAN

Chan is a 42-year-old man who lives with his wife and two children (aged 10 and 8) in a semi-detached house in a rural community. Following a stroke involving the middle cerebral artery in the non-dominant hemisphere, Chan has been referred to the local rehabilitation unit. Chan has had raised blood pressure for 3 years and has been attending regular appointments with his GP but has not followed any advice given in relation to his lifestyle. As a result of the stroke Chan has a left-sided weakness of his left arm and leg.

Changes in body functions and structure

Chan has a change in the functions of his left arm and leg. There has been a change in structure in terms of a bleed into the brain.

Activities and participation

Capacity

- Before the stroke Chan was independent in all activities of daily living. Since the stroke, Chan has the capacity to be independent in most activities of daily living if his clothes are adapted, if his bed is at the right height and if he showers rather than having a bath. Chan is able to walk unaided with the help of a walking aid but he needs assistance with stairs.

Performance

- In terms of actual performance Chan is not able to dress himself without assistance. He needs help to get in and out of bed.
- This difference between capacity and performance is due to Chan's lack of confidence in his abilities. When Chan returns home the physical environment may affect his performance.

Environmental factors

- Chan lives in a close community with supportive neighbours and friends. Already they have been supporting Chan's wife and the children.
- Chan is the only driver in his family and the car is a necessary means of transport. There is a limited bus service.
- In terms of his home environment, the toilet and bathroom are upstairs, as is Chan's bedroom. There are steps leading into the house and into the back garden.
- Chan's employers are not keen for him to return to work as they are concerned that he will not be able to fulfil his work role and that there may be health and safety issues. They are also not open to Chan returning to work in a part-time role.

Personal factors

- Chan has been the main wage earner in his family, with his wife looking after the house and his children. This is an important role for a man in Chinese culture. Chan feels that he has lost the respect of his wife and family because he is unable to resume this role at present.
- Chan's children are having difficulty relating to him. Chan was always playing with his children but because he is not able to resume that role at present he finds it difficult to relate to them.
- Chan and his wife enjoyed a physical relationship before his stroke. Since his stroke his wife is afraid to touch him in case she hurts him and Chan feels he is a lesser man and that his wife won't want him any more.
- In the past, Chan and his wife always talked over any problems and issues. This was their way of coping. Since the stroke they have not really talked about the situation and the future.

CASE STUDY MYRTLE

Myrtle is a 75 year old West Indian woman who lives in a nursing home. She was a health-care assistant working nights for 40 years in a community hospital, retired at 65 and has six children and 12 grandchildren. Five years ago Myrtle's husband died unexpectedly of a heart attack. Myrtle found it hard to cope without him, despite the support of her children. Two years ago Myrtle fell at home and fractured her right neck of femur. She made a good recovery from this; however, she and her family agreed that it would be better if she moved to a nursing home. They were particularly concerned about Myrtle's poor eyesight and lapses of concentration, which had caused her fall at home. Since being in the nursing home Myrtle has had a number of falls, which have again been due to lapses of concentration and poor eyesight. Myrtle does have glasses but forgets to wear them. Two weeks ago she fractured her left neck of femur and is now back in the nursing home having physiotherapy.

Changes in body functions and structure

In terms of body functions there has been a change in the function of Myrtle's left leg and in the functioning of her eyes, this is due to the change in body structure in terms of her fracturing her left femur. There may also be a change in the structure of her eyes that is affecting their functioning. Although not proven there may be some changes in structure and function that may account for Myrtle's lapses of concentration and poor memory.

Activities and participation

Capacity

- Before she fractured her left neck of femur Myrtle was able to look after herself in terms of self care. She joined in with the social activities of the home. Since the fracture Myrtle is beginning to walk with the physiotherapist. She does have the capacity to wash and dress herself but she needs help with putting on her lower garments. Myrtle is not able to bath on her own.

Performance

- In terms of actual performance Myrtle will not wash and dress herself. She continually asks for assistance.
- This difference between capacity and performance is due to Myrtle taking on the 'sick role', not wanting to get out of bed or perform any self-care activities for herself.
- Myrtle's memory may also affect her performance in that she is unable to remember what people have told her.

Environmental factors

- The physical environment of the nursing home has in the past not caused any problems for Myrtle. She is on the ground floor, sharing a room with another female resident that has its own toilet and shower. There is also a communal bathroom for residents. However, since this latest fracture, sharing a room has been causing distress both to Myrtle and to her room-mate. Myrtle calls for the nurses constantly, either by call bell or by shouting out.

Personal factors

- Myrtle has always been a lady of 'strong character'. She has been the strong one of the family, taking control of family events, being 'advisor' to her children.
- Since her husband's death Myrtle has taken on a more passive role, wanting to be told what to do.

CASE STUDY SHELLY

Shelly is 27 and works for a law firm in the city. She graduated with a first class honours degree from her university and is considered a 'high flyer' in her field. Her family are living in Canada and she travels to see them frequently. She has a wide circle of friends and for the past year has been seeing Jonathan, who works for the same firm. It was while she was on a winter sports holiday in Europe with Jonathan that she had a skiing accident, which left her with spinal cord injuries. As a result of this she has a spinal cord lesion at T10. After spending some time in a European hospital while her condition was stabilised, she has now flown back to a spinal injuries unit, where she has been receiving rehabilitation. The team working with Shelly have noticed her becoming more and more withdrawn since her admission, and she has been talking to them about how hopeless she feels and that she wishes her life would end.

Changes in body functions and structure

In terms of structure Shelly has an injury to her spine, which has caused a change in the functions of her legs. She is paralysed from the waist down. There is also some change in bladder function, which means that Shelly doesn't always know when she needs to urinate.

Activities and participation

Capacity

- Before the accident Shelly was independent in all activities of daily living. Since the accident she has the capacity to be independent in an electric wheelchair, using a transferring board to move from chair to bed. She is continent of urine generally but still has the occasional accident. She is able to change her own clothes.

Performance

- Shelley's actual performance is hindered by her depression. She finds it hard to motivate herself to be self-caring and also to take an interest in her personal affairs. This has resulted in her needing help in washing, dressing and transferring. When she is incontinent of urine it is generally because she doesn't have the motivation to get to the toilet in good time.

Environmental factors

- Shelly has not been able to return to her flat because of problems with access. She wants staff and her family to tell her what to do and she relies on Jonathan to deal with her personal affairs.

Personal factors

- Shelly has always been a sociable person with a wide circle of friends. She liked trying new experiences and enjoyed being active, participating in different sports.
- Shelly was ambitious in terms of her job. She liked challenges and needed to feel in control of her life.

Looking at the case studies it can be seen how using the ICF can help create a more complete picture of an individual, considering more than just their disabilities. The identification of personal factors can enable professionals to see what the implications of these are for the individual's function in terms of physical and psychological. This is highlighted in the case of Shelly in that it is the psychological aspects that are affecting her physical function.

It is interesting that in all of the case studies there is a difference in the activities and participation section between capacity and performance. The reasons for this difference are also different in each case study. For Myrtle, taking on the sick role may affect her actual performance. Her reaction may also be because she does not want to be left on her own and in fact her need is to have constant interaction with others. The focus on capacity and performance in the ICF enables this to be recognised; however Wade & Halligan (2003) point out that the ICF doesn't consider how much the individual's choice influences their performance or activities. Chan's performance is affected by his confidence in his abilities, which may also be affected by his environment. Shelly's performance is affected by her lack of motivation, which can be seen as resulting from her depression and feelings of hopelessness.

One of the limitations of the ICF is that it doesn't acknowledge that the individual has a past and a future (Wade & Halligan 2003). All the case studies highlight the influence of time on the individuals.

CONCLUSION

This ICF developed from the ICIDH to encompass changes in thinking about the medical and social model of disability. This move from focusing on disability to focusing on what is important to the individual, considering contextual and personal factors, fits in with the aim of rehabilitation being to optimise the individual's quality of life. This chapter has considered the need for the changes and discussed in more detail the various elements of the ICF. The survey that was carried out, although now a few years old, supports the need for the ICF but also highlights the need for training for professionals to use it.

The ICF is a useful tool for rehabilitation professionals because it provides a common language and also ensures that they are truly taking a holistic view of the client. It could also assist in client-centred goal planning. The ICF needs to continue to develop, as described in the literature, and more research needs to be undertaken as to its usefulness in rehabilitation.

QUESTIONS FOR DISCUSSION

- How can the ICF be used in your team to meet the aims of rehabilitation for individuals?
- How does the ICF fit in with other frameworks you use in practice?
- If you already use the ICF in rehabilitation practice, have you identified any limitations with it and if so how might these be overcome?

References

Bornman J 2004 The World Health Organisation's terminology and classification: application to severe disability. Disability and Rehabilitation 26:182–188

Buckley W 1967 sociology and modern systems theory. Prentice-Hall, Englewood Cliffs, NJ

Chinn PA 1998 Theoretical bases for rehabilitation. In: Chinn PA, Finocchiaro D, Rosebrough A (eds) Rehabilitation nursing practice. McGraw-Hill, New York

Cieza A, Brockow T, Ewert T et al 2002 Linking health-status measurements to the international classification of functioning, disability and health. Journal of Rehabilitation Medicine 34:205–210

Crews JE, Campbell VA 2001 Health conditions, activity limitations, and participation restrictions among older people with visual impairments. Journal of Visual Impairment and Blindness August:453–467

Dahl TH 2002 International classification of functioning, disability and health: an introduction and discussion of its potential impact on rehabilitation services and research. Journal of Rehabilitation Medicine 34:201–204

Davis S 1995 An investigation into nurses' understanding of health education and health promotion with a neuro-rehabilitation setting. Journal of Advanced Nursing 21:951–959

Davis S, O'Connor S 2004 Rehabilitation nursing: foundations for practice, 4th edn. Baillière Tindall, Edinburgh

De Kleijn-de Vrankrijker MW 2003 The long way from the International Classification of Impairments, Disabilities and Handicaps (ICIDH) to the International Classification of Functioning, Disability and Health (ICF). Disability and Rehabilitation 25:561–564

Goodall C 1995 Is disability any business of nurse education? Nurse Education Today 15(5):323–327

Gray DB, Hendershot GE 2000 The ICIDH-2: developments for a new era of outcomes research. Archives of Physical Medicine and Rehabilitation 81(2):10–14

Heerkens Y, van der Brug Y, Ten Napel H et al 2003 Past and future use of the ICF (former IDICH) by nursing and allied health professionals. Disability and Rehabilitation 25:620–627

Hoeman S 1996 Rehabilitation nursing: process and application, 2nd edn. CV Mosby, St Louis

Hurst R 2003 The international disability rights movement and the ICF. Disability and Rehabilitation 25:572–576

Hymovich DP, Hagopian GA 1992 Chronic illness in children and adults: a psychological approach. W B Saunders, Philadelphia

Jette AM, Haley SM, Kooyoomjian JT 2003 Are the ICF activity and participation dimensions distinct? Journal of Rehabilitation Medicine 35:145–149

Kearney PM, Pryor J 2003 The International Classification of Functioning, Disability and Health (ICF) and nursing. Journal of Advanced Nursing 46:162–170

Kielhofner G 2002 Model of human occupation, 3rd ed. Lippincott Williams & Wilkins, Baltimore

King IM 1981 A theory for nursing: systems, concepts, process. John Wiley, New York

Leddy S, Pepper JM 1989 Conceptual bases of professional nursing. JB Lippincott, Philadelphia

Maslow AH 1968 Toward a psychology of being, 2nd edn. Van Nostrand-Reinhold, Princeton, NJ

Neuman B 1982 The Neuman Systems Model: applications to nursing education and practice. Appleton-Century-Crofts, Norwalk, CT

Ogonowski JA, Kronk RA, Rice CN et al 2004 Inter-rater reliability in assigning ICF codes to children with disabilities. Disability and Rehabilitation 26:353–361

Orem D 1985 Nursing – concepts and practice, 3rd edn. Prentice-Hall, London

Parenboom RJM, Chorus AMJ 2003 Measuring participation according to the international classification of functioning, disability and health (ICF). Disability and Rehabilitation 25:577–587

Post MWM, deWitte LP, Schrijvers AJP 1999 Quality of life and the ICIDH: towards an integrated conceptual model for rehabilitation outcomes research. Clinical Rehabilitation 13:5–15

Rentsch HP, Bucher P, Dommen-Nyffeler I et al 2003 The implementation of the international classification of functioning, disability and health (ICF) in daily practice of neurorehabilitation: an interdisciplinary project at the Kantonsspital of Lucerne, Switzerland. Disability and Rehabilitation 25: 411–421

Roy C 1984 An introduction to nursing: an adaptation model, 2nd edn. Prentice Hall, Englewood Cliffs, NJ

Stucki G, Ewart T, Cieza A 2002 Value and application of the ICF in rehabilitation medicine. Disability and Rehabilitation 24:932–938

Universal Declaration on the Human Genome and Human Rights 1997 United Nations, New York. Available on line at http://www.ohchr.org/english/law/genome.htm

Wade DT 2001 Social context as a focus for rehabilitation. Clinical Rehabilitation 15:459–461

Wade DT, Halligan P 2003 New wine in old bottles: the WHO ICF as an explanatory model of human behaviour. Clinical Rehabilitation 17:349–354

World Health Organization 1980 The international classification of impairments, disabilities and handicaps. World Health Organization, Geneva

World Health Organization 2001 International classification of functioning, disability and health. World Health Organization, Geneva

SECTION 2

Models and theories

Chapter 3

Models – terminology and usefulness

Kevin Reel, Sally Feaver

INTRODUCTION

The aims of this chapter are:
- To explore and define the terms associated with conceptual models
- To identify the relationship between these concepts
- To discuss the potential benefits of applying a model to guide practice
- To consider the use of models from the perspective of an individual client.

This chapter will look at the terminology associated with conceptual models, and the muddle that seems to characterise the writing on the subject. This muddle stems in part from the differing definitions of concepts such as frames of reference, treatment approaches, theories and models. There is divergence or disagreement arising within each individual profession (McKenna 1994, Pedretti & Early 2001); thus, when bringing a team of different professionals together, it may seem an insurmountable challenge to gain even a modicum of agreement between them all. For the practitioner, frustration and a sense of professional isolation can result – but for the client, the effect could well be more serious.

While attempting to clarify what we understand to be the relationship between these concepts, we will also consider some of the potential benefits that accrue from the application of a conceptual model to guide practice, both for the client and for the professional. In elaborating our use of the terms it is likely that we will use some of them differently from, even contradictorily to, other writers. While this is unfortunate, the most important outcome is awareness of the different concepts and their contribution to the case we wish to make in favour of the use of conceptual models. The semantic debate is most probably intractable; it is the engagement in it that is important.

Shelly

To put this discussion into context, let us consider briefly the situation of Shelly who was introduced in Chapter 2. She has had a traumatic injury to her spine and is now on an unfamiliar journey through the maze that is acute care followed by rehabilitation. Shelly's day is now filled by many professionals involved in all aspects of her everyday life, from intimate aspects of her self-care through to her functioning as an individual in her broader societal context. The challenge facing the team is to enable Shelly to experience this intervention as cohesive, congruent and meaningful – and clearly progressing toward her short- and long-term goals.

THE RANGE OF KNOWLEDGE, THEORIES, AND IDEAS BEHIND REHABILITATION WORK

We present here our attempt to define and relate the different terms and concepts into a hierarchy of sorts but also to suggest that a linear hierarchical arrangement does not capture the full picture.

A wide range of terms are regularly used when discussing models and practice in general:

- Frames of reference
- Domains
- Treatment approaches
- Paradigms
- Perspectives
- Models
- Philosophies
- Techniques.

The order in which they are listed is not intended to signify anything here, merely to identify some of the terms we will be discussing. After having discussed them, we will offer one view on their relationships to each other.

But first, let's put the terms aside and return to Shelly.

In our interactions with Shelly a variety of ideas and information have a bearing. Some of these have solid theoretical foundations; others are less clear, perhaps only partly relevant or applicable, or perhaps implicit and infrequently verbalised.

If we start at the end, we have a notion of where Shelly wants to get – probably to a satisfying level of participation in her life roles. However straightforward this may seem, this simple notion is informed by a complex array of 'concrete' factual knowledge (e.g. anatomy, physiology) and less 'concrete' but still rigorously derived knowledge (e.g. psychology, sociology). This array influences the way we think about what outcomes are possible in the first instance, and then about how we work with Shelly to achieve them. These make up the hard 'objective' science behind what we do.

There is yet another realm of thought influencing our goals – a set of beliefs or principles about things like the value of independence, the right of the individual to be enabled to achieve that independence, and even about the manner in which we do our work. This could be seen as the more subtle 'subjective' underpinnings that inform our practice. In this realm are values (or philosophical principles) such as respect for human dignity, self-actualisation and autonomy, equality of rights to care and services and the importance of client-centred practice. More recent additions to this realm, at least explicitly so, are values such as continuing professional development, evidence-based practice and reflective practice. An example of an emergent value is the notion of governance – a constant striving for the best and most efficient practice in client care and research.

These core philosophical beliefs are brought to every interaction with clients, in any context. They are not specific to particular clients or particular contexts. Indeed, if they are questioned in a particular situation, this is a philosophical/ethical challenge – for example providing rehabilitation to someone injured while committing a violent crime. Such a case can give rise to a conflict between the principles supporting equitable access to care and the idea that someone injured through no 'fault' of their own might warrant a higher priority if care must be rationed in any way.

The solid underpinnings are sometimes shared between professions, sometimes specific to them. For example, principles of the structure and function of connective tissue will inform the care and treatment of Shelly's now paralysed lower limbs for all staff working with her, but the principles of joint mobilisations might only be employed by the physiotherapist. The same is true for the other ideas. While all care professionals might be aware of the relevance of social networks to Shelly's achievement of her goals, it might be that the domain of one profession's practice brings more specific elements of this realm of knowledge to their work with her.

A profession-specific philosophy would be subscribed to by all practitioners within a particular discipline, but again this would underpin practice with all clients across all settings, for example 'clients' right to be treated with dignity' – largely a tacit assumption, unspoken, unasserted but thoroughly internalised. So embedded might this principle be that its existence is made apparent only when one suffers an affront to this assumption. For example, our reaction to the news stories of former Eastern Block hospitals where people were treated with little dignity – using caged beds to restrain patients – throws such fundamental philosophical assumptions into clear relief (Goldsmith 2004).

In profession-specific ways, certain philosophies underpin certain fields – for example, while all would consider functional ability to be a priority, this focus is the hallmark of occupational therapy, where Shelly's individual ability to carry out the functions and occupations important to her would be the thrust of any intervention.

Against the backdrop of these philosophical assumptions, and in keeping with the most up-to-date knowledge base of relevant subjects, we then use one or more organised 'clusters' of information to make individual decisions about interventions with particular clients. These 'clusters' are commonly called frames of reference or treatment approaches (and sometimes referred to as models, although not the conceptual models we will discuss later). Examples of such 'clusters' are developmental, biopsychosocial, cognitive, behavioural, musculoskeletal. Each of these is associated with an amalgamation of information about how and why things work the way they do. This amalgamation is a contained one – defining a certain approach or perspective that should only be taken to illuminate part of Shelly's whole story. We would not consider it good practice to consider Shelly's mind in isolation from her body, or vice versa. This would be patently simplistic. Such a simplistic view was the hallmark of a divided or dualist approach – seeing the mind and body as separate entities and therefore dealt with separately. This led to what is called reductionism, where one viewed the challenges (at least in physical medicine) as damaged bits that required only the appropriate intervention. While this is frequently described as the medical model, we would suggest this to be a misnomer for a number of reasons. Firstly, there are plenty of practitioners other than medical ones who could be deemed to employ a reductionist perspective. Secondly, there are plenty of medical practitioners who find such an approach to medicine wholly inadequate. And thirdly, it is not really a 'model' in the sense we understand the term. It more closely resembles a perspective on disease or disability, or perhaps a paradigm. It evolved from an ethos in the scientific world suggesting that pretty much everything could be clearly studied and understood, and then manipulated to some degree (albeit within certain boundaries). Time and experience have proved that this approach or perspective is insufficient for most interventions in cases of complex health and social care (Barbour 1995, Longino & Murphy 1995, Medical Research Council 2000).

So we choose the relevant approaches or frames of reference according to the client and their situation – the nature of which challenges and affects the goals they set for their rehabilitation. From that point we then choose the individual techniques we use to achieve those goals, given the other factors.

If we consider Shelly again, we start from a philosophical standpoint that sees her as an autonomous individual with a right to the necessary available assistance to achieve her goals in rehabilitation. We then consider the relevant areas of knowledge useful to the work of achieving those goals. As we take a holistic approach, that range of knowledge is wide and varied. We then consider the principles for treatment arising from that knowledge – the approaches we might use. These may be influenced by a particular frame of reference, or a number of them. At that point, we choose the appropriate techniques suggested by those approaches or frames of reference.

TERMS DEFINED

Having considered them contextually, we now return to our list of terms to explore some more formal explanations and definitions.

Philosophical assumptions

Different professional groups will have philosophical beliefs that focus attention on particular aspects of problem resolution. In its broadest sense, Craig (1983) defined philosophy as:

the study which reveals to us the meaning of existence, the nature of real-ity and our place in it. A philosophy is a creed, a set of beliefs to live by; it provides a purpose encompassing and overriding the minor and triv-ial concerns of the everyday, or if not, it communicates a state of mind from within which the ultimate purposelessness of life becomes endurable.

Where professionals are thinking about the fundamental underpinnings of how and why they do what they do, philosophy is focused more pre-cisely, although it retains its somewhat profound nature. Craig suggested that the philosophical assumptions of a profession are the basic beliefs shared by its members. So professional philosophy is the system of beliefs and values unique to each profession, which provides its mem-bers with a sense of identity and exerts control over theory and practice. It helps locate the domains of concern for that profession – irrespective of the particular practice context. An example of an occupational therapy belief is that occupation is a central aspect of the human experience. In any setting, the occupational therapist would work in a way that recog-nises this belief.

It is arguable that all practitioners hold a set of core beliefs that derive from a variety of sources, one of which is their sense of how the work they do 'fits' into the grand scheme of things. Many practitioners might find it a challenge to identify these underpinnings, but that does not diminish their importance. Indeed, it is these quiet assumptions that keep the project of health care continuing day after day. These central convictions generally carry strong notions about people and how they 'tick', and how one helps them 'tick' best.

Shared philosophy   The following are some of the philosophical assumptions that are com-mon to many professions.

Health-care ethics   Basic assumptions such as the duty of care, respect for client autonomy and just distribution of resources are inherent in each profession's code of practice or standards of conduct. While they may be described in a slightly different fashion, they are based on simi-lar principles that are largely shared across all of health care. Although significantly different at first glance, the values underpinning the Four Principles (Gillon 1986, Beauchamp & Childress 2001) are closely aligned with those behind the Ethical Grid (Seedhouse 1998), although the approaches to organising them are different. Fundamental assumptions such as the client's right to be treated with respect and dignity – become apparent in their universality when offended. With few exceptions, most health-care professionals in developed Western countries react with sim-ilar outrage when confronted by images of 'care' that run contrary to those core values and beliefs that underpin their work. The reports of hospitals in former Eastern block countries using cages and heavy seda-tion to manage individuals with mental health problems is an example of an affront to shared fundamental convictions about dignity and respect for persons and the sensitive nature of any decision to curtail autonomy.

Client-centred practice   Health care that is tailored to the individual as far as possible, approached as a partnership where appropriate and focusing on the goals of the client themselves has become the standard conception of intervention in contemporary settings.

An important point in the context of the professional debate about terms and models is that, from the client's perspective, professional terminology is largely irrelevant, probably just nonsensical semantics.

Shelly has experienced an assault on her life's unfolding narrative; she has had a traumatic derailment. What Shelly experiences are day-to-day difficulties and hopes that these will improve. She may well experience a sense of integrated care from many professionals when the team's work is coordinated under an overarching model. The particularly complex nature of the rehabilitation context makes this most important, the benefits more pronounced. Thus it is essential that the client is spared our debates and disagreements. These must be addressed as constructively as possible outside the client's sphere, leaving only the experience of a cohesive team effort toward realising Shelly's goals.

Developmental/lifelong context   The timeline of Shelly's life is long and continuous – the health-care workers need to understand and appreciate the entirety of it, not simply the current episode they encounter at the point of their involvement. For Shelly, the developmental context now includes the process of rehabilitation and adaptation. Shelly's life narrative has been unexpectedly redirected but the need to see the entirety of it remains.

Profession-specific philosophy

Within each profession, these notions take specific angles. Writing from an occupational therapy perspective, we see occupation (defined in a particular way) as the focus when engaging with Shelly. Other disciplines might hold their own 'primary' philosophy in addition to the shared ones.

Shared knowledge base (and subsequent theory)

There is shared professional knowledge that is used by all health-care professionals, which provides theoretical perspectives on intervening to assist clients with meeting the challenges they face. Biomedical sciences, psychology and sociology are all part of the shared knowledge base that is not profession-specific but used by all health- and social-care professionals. A common understanding of human physiology leads us to develop certain expectations for Shelly's progress in terms of her physical rehabilitation. However, the same knowledge base can be organised differently, in keeping with the focus of the profession. Nursing may adopt a homeostasis perspective; physiotherapy might be more concerned with motor control, strength and range of motion, while occupational therapy might use the same information to guide approaches to energy conservation and work simplification in activities of daily living. In adopting such perspectives for professional roles, knowledge is arranged into theoretical systems or frameworks, which give rise to intervention. A theoretical framework consists of a description of a set of phenomena, an explanation of how and under what circumstances they occur and a demonstration of how they relate to each other. A theory is not 'reality' per se but a structure invented to guide, control or shape it in order to achieve some particular purpose. Theories are constructed out of available knowledge – not as an intellectual exercise but for a purpose. As the purpose varies, so too does the structural complexity of the theory. A good theory will fulfil the purpose for which it was developed. Sociological theory may provide some understanding of Shelly's health/illness beliefs and how she may engage with her recovery.

Other examples of theories used in conceptual models include theories of human development, learning theory, theories of occupation and general systems theory.

Frames of reference

Compatible theories can be organised into frames of reference. A frame of reference, as defined here, consists of a group of compatible theories that can be applied within a particular field of practice. This means that any profession may use a variety of frames of reference.

Frames of reference are clusters of theories selected or developed by different professionals out of the need to support the philosophical beliefs that are the core of the profession. Theories that are not compatible with professional beliefs are not adopted. The theories that are identified as making up the professional body of knowledge arise from and support the philosophical assumptions of the individual profession. For example, behavioural frames of reference may not be part of the frame of reference used by art therapists. Each of the professions uses frames of reference to achieve their unique goals for rehabilitation.

Frames of reference give principles on which to base specific intervention. Frames of reference are aimed at specific problems and professionals choose from a number of appropriate frames of reference.

Examples of frames of reference commonly used in mainstream health and social care settings are biomechanical, psychodynamic, neurodevelopmental, educational, behavioural and rehabilitation.

Selecting frames of reference

Hurff (1985) suggested that the choice of a particular frame of reference is influenced by the challenges faced by the client, the philosophical assumptions of the institutional/organisational context and the experience and bias of the therapist.

Frames of reference are selected using clinical reasoning skills; the criteria for selection include the nature of the condition, the context of the treatment setting and the particular specialism of the health professional. They are part of the shared knowledge between professional groups. Rehabilitation is a good example of a shared frame of reference. All professionals working in a rehabilitation context would be expected to share an understanding of the common underlying principles and base their intervention (interdisciplinary or profession-specific) on these principles. One of these principles might be the idea that some recovery will occur but residual problems will remain; thus, intervention options need to include modification of the environment, adaptation of the tasks and compensation for unrecoverable capacities.

Frames of reference do not always mix well; indeed some would seem to be incompatible. For example, when a person is working to improve their mobility, a neurodevelopmental or normal movement frame of reference may lead to an approach that prefers gait analysis and retraining. A rehabilitation frame of reference might favour the introduction of a walking aid in order to enable the client to achieve functional walking and participation sooner, rather than more 'normal' walking later.

Techniques

The frames of reference give rise to treatment approaches and subsequent intervention techniques. These may be shared or specific. Examples of techniques that are often profession-specific are stoma care, catheter care, respiratory aspiration, wheelchair assessment and pressure care.

Paradigms versus models

One of the sources of confusion in this literature is simply the different terms used for the same concepts and none more so than the term 'model'. Mosey (1981) used the 'model' to refer to the internal structure and content of the profession as a whole, i.e. the typical way in which a profession perceives itself and its relationship to the context in which it operates. Fawcett (2003) paraphrases the rejection of a nursing model as 'they are contributing to the extinction of the discipline of nursing'.

However, Creek (1990) referred to this overview of the structure, content and purpose of a profession as the profession's paradigm. The term 'paradigm' was originally used by Kuhn (1962) to refer to 'coherent traditions of scientific research' and was adopted by Kielhofner & Burke (1977) to refer to 'a dynamic model of bodies of knowledge that demonstrates how they develop, exist, and guide the efforts of professionals'. For many nurses and therapists, 'paradigm' has come to mean the profession's world view. The importance of this discussion is simply to understand the way in which new material starts to influence the way in which professions adopt new concepts. Much has been written about the manner in which new paradigms are rejected or accepted. This seems to take place in such a way that a measured transition is not apparent, but rather there is a complete rejection of the old and a total acceptance of the new. Sometimes there is resistance and oscillation between the two, but it often seems like an all-or-nothing decision for the individual practitioner or theorist. Eventually, where the new paradigm is sound, the tide of opinion in the profession in general might turn. This is a useful concept as it helps us understand how commonly accepted views change personally and professionally.

So far, we have given a brief outline of two sets of knowledge. One is often implicit, the underlying 'softer' type – paradigms and philosophies. The other is that which derives from the 'hard' science pursuits – biology, anatomy, physiology and even psychology and sociology – the frames of reference, treatment approaches and intervention techniques.

The latter is sometimes internalised, but it is often concrete and observable – it guides what we do with Shelly; 'why' in the science sense, 'how' in the practical sense. The former we carry with us and manifest in a more subtle internalised fashion for the most part – it guides 'why' in the existential sense and, in some respects, 'how' in the interpersonal sense.

So where is the model connection? Firstly, there is a distinction to make. Here we refer to models as 'conceptual models'. It is often the case that writers use the term model to refer to treatment models (meaning frames of reference sometimes, and treatment approaches at other times). This is, in part, where some of the muddle around understanding models creeps in. So here, 'model' is meant to be understood as conceptual model.

Remembering the broader contexts – part of our paradigms

In exploring these debates, it is important to remember that the discussion is clearly limited by our particular contexts – practice that is largely happening in affluent Western societies. This context is one that affords the luxury of devoting time and energy to these debates and the development of theoretical constructs within a climate of client-centred practice, enablement and a rights-based approach to civil society. Other factors such as clinical governance and the 'consumer identity,' increasingly encouraged among the public, have their impact as well, as does the market (or pseudo-market) economy in which health care has been set for many years now in many developed countries.

Conceptual models

What is a conceptual model? In general language a model is an organising tool designed to assist in categorising ideas and structuring approaches to help people to make sense of complex phenomena.

Fawcett (2003) sees a conceptual model as made up of concepts (words describing mental images) and propositions (statements expressing the relations between concepts). A conceptual model therefore is defined as a set of concepts and the statements that explain their interrelation in a simplified fashion.

The rise of conceptual models throughout health care

Therapy and nursing in the UK have always been primarily practical disciplines. They have historically tended to show more interest in extending their practical skills and techniques than in developing professional theory. This skills focus is not something to be derided – it is essentially a reflection of the client-centred 'hands on' nature of the work.

At the same time, there is a drive towards health-care practice becoming increasingly evidence based. Many areas of practice involving rehabilitation are, however, far from exact sciences and there is a wide range of knowledge upon which interventions are based. Some of this is shared, some of it is profession-specific. Each of these professions uses the relevant knowledge base to inform their practice. Each has their own role and function to play in the programme of interventions offered to the client.

Over the past decades, however, there has been increasing interest in the use of conceptual models for practice. This interest has taken the form of critiquing existing models, adapting them and developing entirely new models.

Contributing to this in the last two decades in the UK has been the move from professional training into higher education degree level qualification, which has fuelled a plethora of articles and debates within the nursing arena – one of which is the use of nursing models – as the profession responds to the technological change in health care. Practitioners are increasingly asked to produce, identify and/or make use of evidence in order to justify their practice. Although an overall aim of enhancing practice is evident, again this tension between practice and theory sparked debate about the extent to which this endeavour is genuinely aimed at improving client care, or fundamentally concerned with advancing professional status. This tension is a healthy one, keeping the two valid aims in view at all times. The relationship between theory and practice must be a dynamic and interactive one – neither being sustainable without the other.

Why bother with a model when working with Shelly?

Kielhofner (1992) suggested that a model 'elevates clinical practice from a simple application of techniques to a professional process of conceptual problem solving, planning and action'. While this 'elevation' of our work is something that should be sought after by professionals in order to maintain an appreciation of the complexity of their work, it is also of great benefit to the client. This benefit takes the form of not just a successful outcome for their rehabilitation but also a successful, more rewarding collaborative process along that path. In health care generally there is an increasing emphasis on interprofessional working – this has become a priority and is now extending to the development of interprofessional education for health-care workers at all levels, both pre- and postqualifying.

Rehabilitation is one of the areas of practice in which there are many different professionals working with people with problems affecting all areas of their lives. In this context of complex challenges and equally complex interventions, the importance of effective interprofessional working is clear. Jackson & Davies (1995) describe a further plane of team working – the transdisciplinary team. However, the extent to which even interprofessional or interdisciplinary working is currently being achieved is uncertain. More commonly, good multidisciplinary working might be the norm.

Reforms of the last decades in undergraduate education of health-care professionals have helped progress this aim. However, the reality remains one in which individual professional statutory bodies dictate their own curriculum benchmarks and continue to define the parameters of their profession's practice domains and knowledge base.

The model muddle

This book is clearly premised on the idea that models of practice are useful tools in the delivery of health care to clients like Shelly. There is potential for conceptual models to guide and improve the development and application of practice skills, but also potential to make professional roles and identities clearer to all – clients, colleagues and stakeholders. As the development of, and even more the use of, conceptual models is still in many respects a nascent endeavour, there remains confusion and disagreement about what is meant by a model and what its functions might be for these practical professions. Further confusion arises when considering the relationship between models and other constructs such as frameworks, approaches, theories, concepts and perspectives.

The lexicon for debating these issues is not usually held in common within any individual profession; the confusion is made more complex by a context such as rehabilitation where numerous professions are working together with each client.

While these debates have until more recently been conducted mainly in the academic domain, the care they are meant to frame and guide is implemented in practice and experienced at client level. Thus it is essential that the client is not on the receiving end of this confusion (and sometimes outright disagreement) and particularly important that they are not in any way a pawn in the quest for professional autonomy and the securing of a place within the academic hierarchy that has become a pervasive part of health-care education and provision during the last decade.

However, while the terms may not be shared or defined in the same way, many of the concepts and sensibilities behind them are recognisable to all. To all, that is, except one member of the team – the client. Thus it is paramount that we attempt to understand the value of coordinating our work and making explicit the means by which we aim to achieve our collective ends. Many team members working within a single conceptual model could help with this challenge; at the very least, we need to have an understanding of one another's models and attempt to harmonise the terminology we use with each other and with clients like Shelly. The interactions with Shelly need also to be jargon-wary – using common jargon that is readily explicable might be useful, while avoiding jargon that is either complex or unnecessarily 'professionalises' the discussion of rehabilitation.

Components of a good model for practice

Theorists also seem to agree on what should be included in a good model for practice. A good model identifies what is believed about the nature of people and participation, the way that elements of that nature enable function or lead to dysfunction and non-participation, and how one moves from a situation of dysfunction to one of fuller participation. For example, a behavioural model would be based on the belief that human behaviour is the observable output of the integrated function of the central nervous system. This model will be underpinned by theories of human development, the conditions required for that development to take place and the difficulties that arise from problems or inadequacies in either.

Fawcett (2003) asserts that the credibility of the conceptual model requires evidence of its social utility, social congruence and social significance – i.e. is it right for the time? Does it reflect the most current understanding of the relevant structures and their interactions? Does it capture the role(s) of the professional(s) involved?

Critique of models

The influence of the research agenda has given all health-care professionals the tools with which to test, examine and critically appraise. This needs to be extended to models, otherwise they will become closed ideologic systems. This has similarities with paradigms, where it is understood that paradigm shift only occurs after oscillation between the ideas, with considered rejection or acceptance over time.

Some models are designed for generic use with clients with a wide range of problems, others for a narrow area of specialism. Models designed for a narrow area of specialism will have a specific theoretical background and be chosen because that is congruent with the problems identified, e.g. a model designed for health promotion will have a theory relating to health beliefs and an educational process based on and appropriate for those for whom health promotion is required.

The model muddle is evident in part because different professions and different authors in the same professions do not hold similar views on the definition of the concepts, and use different terms for the same concepts. Put simply, a model can be either a 'conceptual model' that defines a professional domain of concern or it can describe a narrow focus of specialism. That narrow focus is also referred to as a frame of reference. Equally the conceptual model defined by a profession is sometimes referred to as a 'professional paradigm'. In our view, there are two common 'levels' of models and it is important to clarify which level is being described. We prefer to reserve the term model for 'conceptual models', such as the Roper Logan & Tierney (1990) model, which attempts to define the nursing domain of concern. This is similar to the Model of Human Occupation (Kielhofner 2002), which describes a domain of concern specific to occupational therapy as opposed to being specific to individual client- or practice-context needs.

This does not mean that, by implication, models are not client-centred. There is an argument that using a model to define practice ensures a client focus, as opposed to a focus on meeting the needs of the institution/local health-care provider, i.e. a focus on discharge and bed access.

Another argument against models is the well rehearsed argument about the novice-to-expert continuum, where it is postulated that as expertise grows so the need grows for structured guiding frameworks to be useful and more intuitive styles of practice emerge (Creek & Feaver 1993 a, b). Is this not really an internalised framework?

Interestingly it appeared that the 'nursing process' may be a good example of a model that was originally designed to define a domain of concern for nursing, was reduced to a 'simplistic process' and began then to constrain and misrepresent the true spirit of the original idea. Similarly the Model of Human Occupation (Kielhofner 2002) was often criticised as being a simplistic diagram – failing to fully represent the important conceptual framework that the author originally intended. The true failing here is to take the simplistic diagram as the full elaboration of the model. In most cases, the diagram is simply a one-dimensional representation of the relationships between concepts. There is always extensive documentation detailing the full meaning behind them.

CONCLUSION

Rehabilitation and medicine are not exact sciences – conceptual models can give order to particular perspectives on the relevant bodies of knowledge. These perspectives can be large or small, shared or profession-specific. Their use, however, does help ensure that Shelly will benefit from a wide body of knowledge and experience from a range of health-care professionals. Paradoxically, the rapid development of high-tech health care and the rise in expectations of clients has meant that we often find ourselves struggling with the tensions between increasing services and increasing scarcity. When the inevitable tensions arise between the needs of the health- or social-care institution/organisation (often dominated by discharge and cost-cutting, best value and evidence-based efficiency) and those of the team and client (the highest-quality care tailored to the individual's needs), the overarching influence of a conceptual model or models to frame practice can help to retain the client focus.

If we return to the general notion of those more concrete 'objective' and subtle 'subjective' arrays of information underpinning practice, these tensions can become manifest as we carry out the priority work: interventions to sort the care and discharge. These interventions are informed directly by that more objective body of knowledge – frames of reference, treatment approaches and techniques. But we may have a strong sense that there are other aspects of the situation to which these more subjective underpinnings draw our attention. This could simply be a wish to take a more holistic approach than our work context allows, or a sense that the care is not as client-centred as we might like.

In such circumstances, a conceptual model can help us remain in touch with these underpinnings while getting on with the interventions – a virtual link or touchstone to the values we hold about the work we do, even if they cannot be acted upon.

Working together with Shelly can be assisted by a model enabling professionals to identify their shared beliefs, knowledge base and principles of intervention while at the same time retaining a clear sense of those that are profession-specific. The sum total should be a focus on assisting Shelly to achieve the fullest participation in her life's new narrative.

QUESTIONS FOR PRACTICE

1. Is there a model in use in your context? Is it explicit or implicit?
2. Do you recognise this as a conceptual model or a treatment model?
3. In your multiprofessional team, to what extent would you consider philosophies to be shared? at variance?

References

Barbour A 1995 Caring for patients: a critique of the medical model. University Press, Stanford CA

Beauchamp TL, Childress JF 2001 Principles of biomedical ethics, 5th ed. Oxford University Press, Oxford

Craig EJ 1983 Philosophy and philosophies. Philosophy 55:189–201

Creek J (Ed) 1990 Occupational therapy and mental health, principles, skills and practice. Churchill Livingstone, Edinburgh

Creek J, Feaver S 1993a Models for practice in occupational therapy: Part 1. Defining terms. British Journal of Occupational Therapy 56:4–6

Creek J, Feaver S 1993b Models for practice in occupational therapy: Part 2. What use are they? British Journal of Occupational Therapy 56:59–62

Fawcett J 2003a Conceptual models of nursing: international in scope and substance? The case of the Roy Adaptation Model. Nursing Science Quarterly 16:315–318

Fawcett J 2003b On bed baths and conceptual models of nursing. Journal of Advanced Nursing 44:229–230

Gillon R 1986 Philosophical medical ethics. John Wiley, Chichester

Goldsmith R 2004 Czech man's week in a cage. Crossing Continents. BBC Radio 4, 8 July. Notes available on line from http://www.bbc.co.uk

Hurff JM 1985 Visualisation: a decisions making tool for assessment and treatment planning. In: Cromwell FS (Ed) Occupational therapy in health care 1:2,5,12 Haworth Press, New York

Jackson H, Davies M 1995 A transdisciplinary approach to brain injury rehabilitation. British Journal of Therapy and Rehabilitation 2:65–70

Kielhofner G 1992 Conceptual foundations of occupational therapy. FA Davis, Philadelphia

Kielhofner G 2002 Model of human occupation, 3rd ed. Lippincott Williams & Wilkins, Baltimore

Kielhofner G, Burke JP 1977 Occupational therapy after 60 years: an account of changing identity and knowledge. American Journal of Occupational Therapy 31(10) 675–89

Kuhn TS 1962 The structure of scientific revolutions. International Encyclopaedia of Unified Science 2(2). University of Chicago Press, Chicago

Longino CF, Murphy JW 1995 The old age challenge to the biomedical model: paradigm strain and health policy. Baywood, Amityville, NY

McKenna HP 1994 Nursing theories and quality of care. Avery, Aldershot

Medical Research Council 2000 A framework for development and evaluation of RCTs for complex interventions to improve health. Medical Research Council, London. Available on line at: http://www.mrc.ac.uk/pdf-mrc_cpr.pdf

Mosey AC (1981) Occupational therapy: configuration of a profession. Raven Press, New York

Pedretti LW, Early MB 2001 Occupational performance and models of practice for physical dysfunction. In: Pedretti LW, Early MB 2001 Occupational therapy: practice skills for physical dysfunction. Mosby, St Louis, p 3–11

Roper N, Logan W, Tierney A 1990 The elements of nursing. Churchill Livingstone, Edinburgh

Seedhouse D 1998 Ethics: the heart of healthcare, 2nd ed. John Wiley, Chichester

SECTION **3**

Models in Practice

Chapter 4

The Canadian Model of Occupational Performance

Mary Kavanagh

INTRODUCTION

The aims of this chapter are:
- To give an overview of the Canadian Model of Occupational Performance (CMOP)
- To look at the history of the development of the model
- To examine how the model is used in practice
- To discuss the theoretical perspectives underpinning the model
- To examine how the model is used in rehabilitation and its relationship to the International Classification of Functioning, Disability and Health
- To explore how the use of the model may promote or hinder interprofessional working.

As set out above, this chapter aims to give the reader an introduction to a specific model of practice used by occupational therapists, namely the Canadian Model of Occupational Performance (CMOP) (Townsend 1997), which was originally developed in Canada and is now used in many other countries. The case study of Shelly, outlined in Chapter 2, will be used here to illustrate the use of the model in practice.

CASE STUDY SHELLY

Shelly is 27 and works for a law firm in the city. She graduated with a first class honours degree from her university and is considered a 'high flyer' in her field. Her family are living in Canada and she travels to see them frequently. She has a wide circle of friends and for the past year has been seeing Jonathan, who works for the same firm. It was while she was on a winter sports holiday in Europe with Jonathan that she had a skiing accident, which left her with spinal cord injuries. As a result of this she has a spinal cord lesion at T10. After spending some time in a European hospital while her condition was stabilised, she has now flown back to a spinal injuries unit, where she has been receiving rehabilitation. The team working with Shelly has noticed her becoming more and more withdrawn since her admission, and she has been talking to them about how hopeless she feels and that she wishes her life would end.

At this point it would be helpful to give a definition of 'occupational performance' to clarify what the term means. As outlined by Townsend (1997) occupational performance 'refers to the ability to choose, organise and satisfactorily perform meaningful occupations that are culturally defined and age appropriate for looking after one's self, enjoying life and contributing to the social and economic fabric of the community' (p. 30).

This is seen by Law et al (1995) as taking place over the person's lifespan and as a dynamic and flowing relationship between the person, the occupations they engage with and the environment in which they carry out these occupations.

HISTORICAL BACKGROUND TO THE MODEL

The model was first introduced in the 1980s, when a Canadian task force, supported by funding from the Canadian Association of Occupational Therapists and the Department of National Health and Welfare, developed what was then called the 'Model of Occupational Performance'. It was first presented to the general occupational therapy world in 1982 and, following various revisions, was renamed the Canadian Model of Occupational Performance in 1997. The initial drivers behind the development of this model were a concern from both inside and outside the profession regarding quality assurance in occupational therapy services (Townsend et al 1990). Concurrently in the USA, the American Occupational Therapy Association generated a series of task forces and committees whose brief was to develop policy statements about generic areas of concern for the profession, including the development of an occupational therapy model that would reflect the domain of occupational performance. Although a slightly different model from the Canadian Model was developed as a result of this work, nonetheless it can be seen that the drivers were there to make the concept of occupational performance central to the work of occupational therapists (Chapparo & Ranka 1997). Both models ultimately drew on earlier work on the Human Occupations Model by Reed & Sanderson (1984), which focused on the interaction between the person, their occupations and the environment in which these were carried out.

As stated above, various changes have been made to the Canadian Model since its first appearance, particularly to the range of environmental factors impacting on the individual: for example, political, economic and legal environments were added in 1993. As occupational therapy practice evolves, so too does the Model, hence the third revision in 1997, which placed at the heart of the model the concept of 'spirituality' (appreciation of the uniqueness of the individual), in order to ensure that the person the therapist is working with remains the focus of occupational therapy intervention. It also re-emphasised the dynamic and interdependent action between all the elements of the model, which are explained more fully below.

The Canadian Occupational Performance Measure (Law et al 1994a,b), which is used as part of the assessment of occupational performance, is also a development of the work of the task force that worked on the

Canadian Model, since it was identified that there was no outcome measure to gauge improvement from start to finish of occupational therapy intervention in the areas of self-care, productivity and leisure that occupational therapy focused on (Law et al 1990, Pollock 1993). Since its inception it has been used in a variety of clinical settings and a number of different countries (Waters 1995, Mew & Fossey 1996, Trombly et al 1998, Bodiam 1999, Healy & Rigby 1999, Norris 1999, Tryssenaar et al 1999, Wressle et al 1999, Sewell & Singh 2001, Chesworth et al 2002, Gilbertson & Langhorne 2000, Clarke 2003). It is considered a valid and reliable outcome measure for occupational therapists using the Canadian Model as their guiding framework (Law et al 1990, Bosch 1995, Toomey et al 1995, McColl et al 2000).

DESCRIPTION OF THE MODEL AND ITS APPLICATION TO THE CASE OF SHELLY

Overall the model looks specifically at the interaction and interrelationship between the *person*, their *environment*, and the *occupations* performed by that person during their lifetime. It takes the perspective that these three aspects are dynamic and therefore the interplay between them is crucial to the extent to which the person is able to engage in all three independently (Townsend 1997).

For example, prior to her accident, Shelly as a person was living independently and able to engage in a whole range of occupations, including self-care, socialising, working and sports. Her environment consisted of a variety of settings: the law firm, her flat, holiday destinations, places of entertainment, basically the whole community setting. Following her injury, Shelly's environment currently consists of the hospital in which she is receiving treatment, and her occupations are limited to attempting basic self-care.

The Canadian Model proposes a framework for the occupational therapist to work with Shelly from four basic aspects: *spirituality*, which occupies the centre space at the heart of the model, and what are called the *physical, cognitive* and *affective components*.

Spirituality

From the perspective of the Canadian Model the term 'spirituality' refers to the uniqueness of every individual a team will work with, regardless of the similarity of their disabilities (Townsend 1997). It therefore prevents the team from focusing purely on the disability rather than on the *person* who has the disability, therefore relying as much on interactive reasoning as on diagnostic reasoning (Fleming 1991). In acknowledging the person's uniqueness, the therapist is appreciating 'their intrinsic value, [and] respecting their beliefs, values and goals, regardless of ability, age, or other characteristics' (Townsend 1997, p. 42).

The model therefore places the person at the heart of the intervention process (Fig. 4.1) and defines the need to fully engage in partnership with the individual to see what occupations are meaningful to them, therefore not making assumptions about what is relevant or not to the person, and certainly not being prescriptive about what they might or might not enjoy and get pleasure out of (Townsend 1997).

Figure 4.1 The Canadian Model of Occupational Performance (with permission from Townsend 1997)

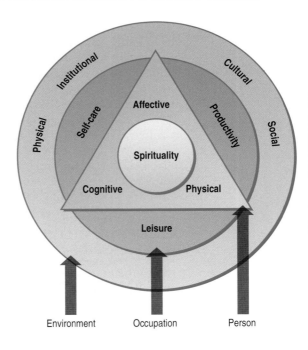

CASE STUDY SHELLY (CONTINUED)

Shelly's parents took her to church regularly when she was a child but Shelly does not consider herself to have any particular religious belief system. She values the individuality of people and tries to treat others with respect. She supports charities such as Oxfam and the Worldwide Fund for Nature, and loves salsa dancing and the theatre and cinema. Considered a charismatic person with a wide circle of friends, she throws herself into activities with a passion. Shelly sees herself as 'always living life to the full', whether travelling, working or meeting up with Jonathan or her friends and family. In terms of her future work and life, Shelly hopes that her relationship with Jonathan will ultimately lead to marriage, and wants children. In the meantime she values her job very highly and wants to travel as much as she can, particularly to Australia and New Zealand.

The physical, cognitive, and affective components

In using the term 'components', the model is referring to the different aspects of function that the person needs in order to engage in occupation. These are grouped into three: *physical*, the 'doing', or the motor, sensory, and sensory motor functions; *cognitive*, the 'thinking' domain, involving both intellectual as well as cognitive functions, including memory, comprehension and reasoning; and *affective*, or the 'feeling' domain, which looks at intrapersonal and interpersonal emotional functions (Townsend 1997). Although these are distinguished here, it is nonetheless important to consider them as interdependent components (Payne & Isaacs 1991), for example when carrying out a task such as dressing, which requires a range of physical function such as fine finger movement, figure ground discrimination, affective function such as desire to engage in the task and cognitive function such as understanding of why the task needs doing and memory of how to put clothes on in the correct sequence.

CASE STUDY SHELLY (CONTINUED)

Physical component (function)

Shelly has a spinal cord lesion at the level of T10, which means that her respiration is unaffected, and she has no movement in her lower extremities. She has the potential to be independent in regulating her bladder and bowel movements and to be able to transfer herself independently. She also should be able to resume driving in a car with adapted hand controls (Pedretti & Early 2001).

Cognitive component (function)

Shelly has only a hazy memory of the accident that led to her injury. She remembers another skier shouting at her to move out of the way, but after that it's a blank. She has been told, and appears to understand, that she has a spinal cord injury and the implications of this. At the moment she finds it difficult to concentrate for long periods as she is easily fatigued, and she is taking analgesics to help control her pain (she sustained some injuries to her arm and face as a result of the accident).

Affective component (function)

Shelly is very low in mood, to the point that she has been diagnosed with clinical depression. She is worried about her job, and whether her firm will continue to employ her now that she has had so much time off work and is disabled as a result of the accident. Her mother Julia has flown over from Canada to be with her, but Shelly is finding it hard to talk to her, as she cries every time she tries to talk about how she is feeling. Most of all she is afraid that Jonathan will no longer want her as she is now disabled, and that she may not be able to conceive a child.

The occupation

The concept of occupation is divided up into the three performance areas of self-care, leisure and productivity. Each performance area is subsequently divided into three subsets to enable therapists to make sure that they cover the broadest range of occupations that an individual might be involved in doing. For example, self-care is divided into: personal care, which includes getting washed and dressed, personal hygiene and eating; functional mobility, which includes transfers, indoor and out; and community management, which includes accessing transportation, shopping and managing finances. Leisure is divided into: quiet recreation, which includes hobbies, crafts and reading; active recreation, such as sports, outings and travel; and socialisation – visiting, parties, phone calls, correspondence. The final area is productivity, which is divided into: work, both paid and unpaid, including all that is involved in finding and keeping a job, also volunteer work; household management, such as cleaning, cooking, and washing; and finally play/school, which consists of play skills and homework (Townsend 1997). In an initial interview, these are the areas that the therapist would concentrate on to get an idea of which specific performance areas the person is having difficulty with and where they need most input in order to maintain or increase their independence. This will be further expanded on in the section dealing with the use of the Canadian Occupational Performance Measure (Law et al 1994a).

As with the section on performance components or functions, the three performance areas are not mutually exclusive, as individuals may need to achieve independence in one area, such as self-care (dressing), before they can engage in productivity or leisure tasks (attending a job interview, dancing). Some activities may also potentially fall into several performance areas, depending on the focus of the task. Cooking, for example, may be classed by the person as a productivity task when it involves feeding a family out of necessity, but may equally be a leisure task when done for pleasure, e.g. making a birthday cake. The choice of which performance area to attribute the task to is up to the individual, not the therapist.

CASE STUDY SHELLY (CONTINUED)

Shelly's occupations currently revolve around basic self-care: dressing her lower body independently; using the toilet and shower on the ward independently; being able to manoeuvre her wheelchair indoors and out; and being able to transfer into/out of a car without help. Through the use of the Canadian Occupational Performance Measure she was able to identify other areas involving productivity and leisure tasks that she set as goals for herself (see below).

The environment

Encircling performance areas and performance components and also intersected by them is the environment, which, as the context in which occupation occurs, can impact positively or negatively on the person's ability to carry out necessary tasks of daily living. It is divided up into a range of categories to encompass the attributes an environment consists of. The *physical environment* contains built surroundings such as houses, car parks, office blocks, transportation (planes, trains, buses, cars). The environment also includes *natural environmental surroundings*, such as the weather, and parks, fields, rivers and mountains. There is the *institutional environment*, with its legislation, funding arrangements, accessibility and employment support. Into this context is also placed the *cultural environment*, which includes the ethnic, ceremonial and routine practices of particular groups of individuals; and finally the *social environment*, which focuses on social groupings based on common interests and patterns of relationships that individuals have (Townsend 1997).

CASE STUDY SHELLY (CONTINUED)

Physical environment

Shelly appreciates that at present the physical environment in which she is living (i.e. the hospital) is the one in which she will first need to learn to be independent, and therefore focuses on learning how to manoeuvre her wheelchair through doors and become more adept at transfers. It is also important to her to be independent in terms of transport, and she asks her mother to help her arrange for her car to be specially adapted for a wheelchair user. The challenge of outside the hospital will also face her when she has to consider how accessible her law firm's building and facilities will be, not to mention her flat in the city.

Natural environment

The difficulty of negotiating grass in her wheelchair as opposed to a flat hospital floor brings home to Shelly how much she needs to plan a lot of activities she has previously carried out automatically. She finds that she gets cold more quickly than usual because of not having as much mobility as she used to.

CASE STUDY SHELLY (CONTINUED)

Institutional environment

Through the social worker in the hospital Shelly becomes aware of how much her life has changed now she has become, in society's eyes, a 'person with a disability'. She is given Disability Living Allowance forms to fill in, and looks into getting a wheelchair user's badge for her car. When she is more able to, she starts negotiations with her employers to find out what support she might need should she return to work and the extent of her employers' responsibility towards her under the Disability Discrimination Act 1994.

Social environment

Shelly comes to value the support of her parents, although initially she did not want to see them, Jonathan or her old friends while she was getting used to being in a wheelchair. She wants to present a more independent Shelly to them, as opposed to someone who is always asking for their help.

Cultural environment

Shelly feels very estranged from her normal culture of parties, work and being with Jonathan, and feels very isolated from her normal environment.

So, all the above, that is, the person, the occupation and the environment, provide the arena in which occupational performance takes place. At this point, the part that chronology plays must also be recognised. Some occupational performance may be discarded at particular points of a person's life when the occupation is no longer needed or wanted, e.g. being fed by a parent when young. The process does not stay static but is constantly changing and developing as the needs and demands of the person, the environment and the occupation change. So too will ageing, disability, and environmental change impact upon the extent to which a person can engage in occupational performance over a certain period of time (Townsend 1997).

APPLICATION OF THE OCCUPATIONAL THERAPY PROCESS MODEL

The structure of the Canadian Model, with its emphasis on the person, the environment and occupation, provides an overarching framework that then needs to be applied in the practice situation. Most occupational therapy processes work along the principles of assessment, planning of intervention and evaluation of interventions (Creek 2002), and the Canadian Model is no different. The occupational therapy process model (Fig. 4.2, Box 4.1) developed by Fearing (1993) and Fearing et al (1997) is used as part of the Canadian Model to engage the person in these three basic principles. Some of the key features of this particular process are that it reflects occupational therapy values and beliefs, is action orientated, and evaluates client outcomes using an appropriate outcome measure, appropriate to diverse environments (Fearing et al 1997).

Stage 1: Naming, validating and prioritising occupational performance issues

At this point the occupational therapist meets with the person to look at specific areas of self-care, productivity and leisure identified by the individual as ones they need some help with. It must be said at this point that this assessment process is designed to run alongside others that are being

Figure 4.2 The Occupational Performance Process Model (with permission from Townsend 1997; adapted from Fearing et al 1997)

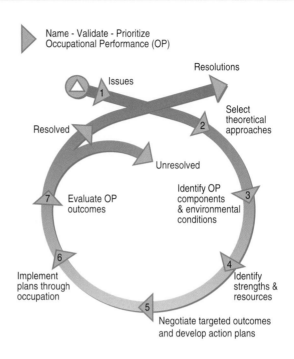

carried out by other members of the multidisciplinary team and that information gathered at this point from the whole team is crucial to the implementation of a holistic and needs-led plan for intervention.

Originally Fearing et al (1997) described the above meeting as one in which to identify 'problem areas' for the person, but the term was deliberately changed to 'issues', a word that was viewed as being emotionally less laden and also respecting the fact that many individuals regard their inability to perform certain activities as less of a problem than a nuisance. The process talks about 'naming, validating and prioritising' issues (Townsend 1997). By this is meant that the therapist asks specific questions to determine precisely what areas of daily living skills the person is

---

Box 4.1   The OT Process Model

The OT process model follows seven stages:
Stage 1:   Naming, validating and prioritising occupational performance issues
Stage 2:   Selecting theoretical approaches
Stage 3:   Identifying occupational performance components and environmental conditions
Stage 4:   Identifying strengths and resources
Stage 5:   Negotiating targeted outcomes and developing action plans
Stage 6:   Implementing plans through occupation
Stage 7:   Evaluating occupational performance outcomes

having some difficulty with, and uses specific listening and feedback skills to determine what the main areas are that need assistance. So for example, a statement that begins with, 'I'm struggling with getting dressed' might through careful questioning be rephrased as, 'I have trouble doing up my buttons because of my arthritis', and therefore the therapist is able to home in on the precise nature of the difficulty. *Validation* means that the therapist acknowledges the person's statement of their difficulties and how important the activity is to them. Finally, by *prioritising*, if many areas are highlighted as important, the therapist can find out which are the most important areas to start working on. Various methods of eliciting this information are suggested, from semi-structured interviews to home visits, as well as the use of the Canadian Occupational Performance Measure (COPM; Law et al 1994a).

The COPM categorises the specific occupational performance areas into self-care, productivity and leisure, and, as above, through focused questioning, the therapist can elicit issues that the person wishes to work on (*naming*) and ask the person to score the importance of these particular tasks out of a score of 1–10, 1 being least important and 10 being the most important (*validating*). After this, in steps 3 and 4 of the measure, the person is asked to choose the five most important areas to work on first (*prioritising*). In these five areas, the person is asked to rate their perspective of their current performance out of 10, 1 being unable to perform the activity and 10 being independent in its performance. They are also asked to rate their level of satisfaction with their current performance of the activity. The COPM is designed as an outcome measure, so that following intervention the initial score may be revisited and it can be seen if there is a difference in scores. This will be developed further, with reference to Shelly, in stage 7.

CASE STUDY SHELLY (CONTINUED)

Shelly's prioritising of her five tasks, and her current performance and satisfaction scores, produced the following:

1. I want to be independent in using the toilet and shower on the ward (Performance 3; Satisfaction 1)
2. I want to be independent in dressing my lower half (Performance 4; Satisfaction 2)
3. I want to be independent in getting around in my wheelchair, both on the ward and in the car park (Performance 3; Satisfaction 1)
4. I want to go out to the cinema with Jonathan (Performance 1; Satisfaction 1)
5. I want to talk to my boss about coming back to work (Performance 1; Satisfaction 1).

Stage 2: Selecting theoretical approaches

With the information provided from stage 1, at this point the therapist needs to look at which theoretical approaches would be the most effective in working with the person. This is influenced by a number of factors: the therapist's knowledge and experience of various interventions, their clinical reasoning skills, their use of supervision, and knowledge of evidence-based practice (Townsend 1997). A number of theoretical approaches or frames of reference may be employed, ranging from health promotion to psychosocial, biomechanical, rehabilitative and educational, depending on the areas identified (Hagedorn 2000).

CASE STUDY SHELLY (CONTINUED)

The occupational therapist has been working on the unit for some time and is experienced in working with individuals with spinal cord injuries. She uses the biomechanical frame of reference to determine what physical function Shelly has, given her lesion at T10. She uses a learning frame of reference, i.e. an educative approach, to help Shelly with problem-solving, the best and most effective way to achieve safe transfers and manoeuvre her wheelchair, and adopt dressing techniques.

The compensatory frame of reference is also used, as some skills and function have been perma-

nently lost, and the therapist therefore helps Shelly develop new techniques and 'trick movements' while transferring, to compensate for lost function. Using a rehabilitative approach, she also provides Shelly with equipment such as a transfer board to enable her to access her car, and explores with Shelly what equipment she would find useful in her flat to help her be as independent as possible. Guiding her whole approach to Shelly is the therapist's use of the humanistic frame of reference, which places the emphasis on Shelly determining her priorities as to how intervention will proceed.

Stage 3: Identifying occupational performance components and environmental conditions

Having identified the performance issues, at this point the therapist needs to talk to the person about what aspects of their physical, cognitive and affective domains are affecting their ability to carry out self-care, leisure and productivity tasks. This may encompass anything from fatigue, poor figure-ground discrimination and memory, to depression, low self-esteem and lack of motivation.

CASE STUDY SHELLY (CONTINUED)

The main factors affecting Shelly are fatigue, pain and her struggle to adjust emotionally to her accident, aside from adjusting to the loss of physical function. She finds her lack of bladder and bowel control particularly embarrassing and, in her eyes, 'demeaning' and

finds it very hard to ask for help. She often has nightmares about the accident, and feels that her mood goes 'up and down'. She asks to see a counsellor on the unit, and also talks particularly to another patient, Lorraine, who has sustained a similar injury.

Stage 4: Identifying strengths and resources

It is important at this point to look at what strengths and resources the person has that may aid the achievement of specific goals already identified. This links in with appreciating the uniqueness of each person and the fact that, although the disability may be similar to another's, each person may have very different resources to help them cope.

CASE STUDY SHELLY (CONTINUED)

In her counselling sessions and also her work with the psychologist on the ward, as well as with the occupational therapist, Shelly is able to look at her strengths and resources and names these as:

- The closeness of her family and Jonathan before the accident
- Her close circle of friends, who are still in contact with her
- The support of her employers, who wish her to return to work
- Her own determination to get well
- Her stubbornness at not accepting defeat
- Her academic and intellectual abilities.

Stage 5: Negotiating targeted outcomes and developing action plans

CASE STUDY SHELLY (CONTINUED)

The occupational therapist works with Shelly to draw up a programme initially focusing on Shelly's goals for independently transferring, and washing and dressing. They set aside time for daily practice, in conjunction with interventions by other members of the team, including the physiotherapist and counsellor, as well as the nursing staff.

Stage 6: Implementing plans through occupation

From all the information gathered from the previous stages, this is where goals can be identified and outcomes set (five) with those plans then being implemented through set targets (six).

CASE STUDY SHELLY (CONTINUED)

Through use of the rehabilitative frame of reference, the therapist works with Shelly daily at the start to give her practice in the above areas until she is able to carry them out first with minimal help and finally independently. She also works with the physiotherapists on the unit to build up her upper limb strength so that she becomes more confident and able to manoeuvre her wheelchair, which leads her on to her next goal of going out with Jonathan to the cinema in his car.

Stage 7: Evaluating occupational performance outcomes

At an agreed date, and again making reference to the COPM, the therapist and the individual together evaluate how the performance issues identified at the start of the intervention have gone up to this point, using the performance and satisfaction rating scale that was originally referred to. If there is no longer an issue with the areas, five new areas from the original list are identified, and if there are outstanding issues still, a re-evaluation of the process continues until all outstanding issues are resolved.

CASE STUDY SHELLY (CONTINUED)

At the agreed date, Shelly and the occupational therapist go through the original goals that Shelly set and look at her current levels of performance and satisfaction. She scores them as follows:

- Independence in toilet and shower. (Performance now 9; Satisfaction 9)
- Independence in dressing lower half (Performance now 10; Satisfaction 10)
- Independence in using wheelchair (Performance now 8; Satisfaction 9)
- Cinema with Jonathan (Performance 10; Satisfaction 7 – mainly due to accessibility issues in the cinema, rather than to issues to do with being with Jonathan).

Shelly has put off speaking to her employers about returning to work as she wants to be in a position where she feels more independent and able to speak from a position where she can be clear about any specific help she may need. Shelly feels that she still needs practice with using her wheelchair, particularly out in public, where she finds kerbs and crossing roads a problem, but feels that she has achieved her goals in the other areas, and therefore chooses four other goals to work on, including getting to her friend's wedding, which is only a month away. She also plans to speak to her employers to fulfil her outstanding goal from the start of her work with the occupational therapist.

THEORETICAL PERSPECTIVES UNDERPINNING THE MODEL

The Canadian Model, as with the Model of Human Occupation (Kielhofner 2002, and Adaptation through Occupation (Reed & Sanderson 1992) are encompassed by the occupational behaviour frame of reference. The focus of the frame of reference supports the development of a balanced range of occupations in a person's life. The focus on occupation as a therapeutic intervention is not new and dates back to the ancient world (Digby 1985), far preceding even the inception of occupational therapy as a profession, as it emerged early in the 20th century. The founders of occupational therapy recognised the health-enhancing effects of carrying out meaningful activities that had purpose for the individual (Peloquin 1991a, b).

As a relatively 'young' profession compared to medicine and nursing, occupational therapy also originally drew on a variety of sources of knowledge, from diverse fields such as psychology, sociology, architecture, anatomy, medicine and psychiatry. This created a rich and diverse pool of knowledge for therapists to draw upon (Creek 2002). During its evolutionary period, therefore, the main emphasis for occupational therapy was on what Hagedorn (2000) termed the 'development of practice', concentrating on the 'what' rather than the 'why' of practice. In the 1980s and 1990s, the profession concentrated much more on developing the rationale for occupational therapy and dwelling on the unique perspective it gives to the purpose of occupation. During that period no fewer than ten models were developed that looked specifically at the interaction between the person, their occupation and the environment (these will be discussed further below).

The main emphasis of the Canadian Model is on the importance of occupation, the uniqueness of the individual and the importance of engaging the individual in determining their own interventions. These will be examined in turn to explore which theoretical perspectives are involved.

The Canadians developed a particular perspective on occupational performance, defining it initially as the therapeutic use of activity in a client-centred framework (Canadian Association of Occupational Therapists 1983). Further beliefs were set out by Townsend in 1997, namely that occupation needs to be seen as a determinant of health, having therapeutic effectiveness, subject to change over a lifetime and, most importantly, giving meaning to life. This philosophy is also shared by other authors (Christiansen & Baum 1997, Wilcock 1998, Kielhofner 2002) and the emerging field of occupational science. Occupational science puts the nature of human occupation and occupational performance at the heart of its academic enquiry (Zemke & Clark 1996) and has been defined as 'the study of the human as an occupational being, including the need for and capacity to engage in and orchestrate daily occupations over the lifespan' (Yerxa et al 1989). So, while complementary to the development of occupational therapy theory, there are nonetheless similarities in what is being said in the context of occupational engagement, or performance, to the Canadian Model. Occupational science also emphasises the value of activity in gaining a sense of identity, the value of learning by doing, and the state of 'flow' that can be achieved by engaging in fulfilling activities (Csikszentmihalyi 1992), which occupational therapists have always recognised (Wright 2004).

The uniqueness of the individual and the need for client–centred practice

The Canadian Model holds that individuals are unique human beings, with intrinsic dignity and worth, able to make choices and with the capacity for self-determination. It also believes that all individuals have the potential to change and have diverse abilities (Townsend et al 1990). This participation in activity also contributes to shaping the person's own sense of self (Christiansen 1999). It therefore is inevitable that, once the individual is recognised as capable of making choices, etc., they should be engaged as partners in the decision-making process, with the focus on client-centred practice. The concept of client-centred practice was a constant theme in the development of the Model, taking its basis from the work of Carl Rogers, who first referred to the term in 1939 in a seminal work entitled *The Clinical Treatment of the Problem Child*. It is rooted in humanistic psychology and has influential theorists, besides Rogers (1986), Frankl (1992), Kelly (1955) and Maslow & Abraham (1987), who placed emphasis on the essentially positive nature of every individual, needing to be valued for themselves. In that way they considered that the individual would respond to this 'positive regard' and be in a position to take control of his or her life. The humanistic view places emphasis on the need for authenticity, honesty and non-judgement (Rogers 1986). Client-centred practice within occupational therapy therefore embraces respect for, and partnership with, all individuals involved in receiving intervention (Townsend 1997) and recognises the strengths that those individuals bring with them, the need they have for choices, and the benefits of collaboration between the person and the individual in planning and implementing goals (Law et al 1995, Sumsion 1999).

SIMILARITIES TO OTHER MODELS

As stated earlier, the period of the 1980s and 1990s saw the development of models whose emphasis was on the person's ability to perform competently their occupations within a physical and social environment (Polatajko 1992, Reed & Sanderson 1992, Stewart 1992, Chapparo & Ranka 1997, Christiansen & Baum 1997, Schkade & Schultz 1997, Hagedorn 2000, Kielhofner 2002).

Hagedorn (2002) terms these the 'occupational performance models' (p.129) and the 'Person-Environment-Occupational Performance (PEOP) models' (*ibid*). All of them have as common values and beliefs similarities with the Canadian Model, in that they view as central the value of occupation as contributing to wellbeing; the uniqueness of the individual; and the person's experience and contribution as vital to the intervention process.

In terms of non-occupational-therapy models, there are some similarities with nursing models, which, while addressing the interaction between the person and their environment, do not specifically talk about occupational performance. However, terms such as adaptation (Roy 1984), self-care (Orem 1985) and activities of daily living (Roper et al 1990) are key concepts for the most common nursing models used in the UK. As well as this, the Illness Constellation Model (Morse & Johnson 1991), which is explored in more detail in Chapter 5, focuses on the experience of wellness, wellbeing and the experience of illness for the individual.

RELATIONSHIP TO REHABILITATION

Occupational therapists have been involved in the process of rehabilitation since their foundation (Creek 2002). The Canadian Model could be considered to work best in areas where therapists have not only the time to build up relationships with the people they are working with, but also the time to work on specific goals. Since the structure of rehabilitation teams consists of clinicians who have a desire to work with individuals over a set period of time to achieve certain outcomes, the Model and the Measure, as already demonstrated above, facilitate this process entirely. Two important tasks identified as being central to the rehabilitation process are the identification of problem areas and goal setting (Wade & de Jong 2000) and the use of the COPM strives to do precisely this.

The emphasis placed by Whiteneck (1994) on the individual receiving treatment being at the heart of the rehabilitation process equally has its echo in the person-centred approach that the Canadian Model, and particularly the COPM, has in enabling the person themselves to identify the areas they perceive as a problem and from that point to participate in identifying with the clinician a strategy for addressing those problem areas. This statement is also backed up by some of the literature already mentioned (Wressle et al 1999, 2001, 2003) and shows that not only does the person participate in goal-setting but that through this process self-esteem and motivation increase, as well as quality of life. This process too relies on a team approach rather than an individual approach, which a rehabilitation setting provides an excellent opportunity for.

Interprofessional working

The research that has taken place concerning the Canadian Model has tended to focus on the use of the COPM and its efficacy as an outcome measure (Law et al 1990, Bosch 1995, Toomey et al 1995, McColl et al 2000). There appears to be little research to date which specifically addresses the use of the Measure as an interprofessional team tool. Fedden et al (1999) implemented the Measure in a community setting for the older person and found that using the Measure enabled them to have a clearer sense of focused communication with the rest of the multidisciplinary team. Their report, however, did not include feedback on how the team perceived the use of the Measure. Wressle et al's study (2003) was conducted in a day-treatment setting in Sweden, the client group having rheumatoid arthritis. Although this involved a relatively small group of clinicians, including occupational therapists, physiotherapists, nurses, social workers and physicians, the overall evaluation by the team of the COPM had some positive results. These included: improved participation from the client perspective, as it specifically involved the latter in the planning of interventions that were specifically meaningful to them. This finding is also supported by an earlier study by Wressle (2002), which looked at the improvement in client participation in the rehabilitation process using the COPM. The other members of the team were also challenged by taking the focus away from function to looking at activity; and finally the team felt that their conferences were affected positively by the structure of the reports that the occupational therapists gave from the results of the COPM, as they clarified the needs of the clients and kept the focus on rehabilitation.

Barriers to interprofessional working

Wressle's (2003) study did highlight some interesting issues about potential barriers to interprofessional working. Although as is stated above, the team were challenged by the emphasis on engagement in activity rather than concentrating on function, which was constraining for team members working primarily from a medical model of care. Here it has to be acknowledged that the Canadian Model is not designed to supersede diagnostic tests or any other interventions that a team would need to carry out. One of the reports from the team was that if they were to do the COPM themselves they would put a different emphasis on questions that they asked of the clients, depending on the perspective they were coming from. This would make sense for them, but in essence would not be true to the purpose of the COPM, with its clear emphasis on performance rather than function.

Similarities and comparisons with the ICF

The International Classification of Functioning, Disability and Health (World Health Organization 2001) has already been covered in some detail in Chapter 2 of this book, so this section proposes only to give a general overview of the former and examine any similarities and differences to the Canadian Model.

The Canadian Model, as with the ICF, is applicable to any individual irrespective of health condition and age. Both also look at the context in which the individual lives and operates, i.e. the environment, in all its forms, and both look at the personal factors, which can enable or disable the person in terms of how able they are to be independent in functioning. The three levels of human functioning as described by the ICF (the level of the body; the whole person; the whole person in a social context) find their counterparts almost completely at the level of the physical performance components; the person; and the environment, as outlined in the Canadian Model.

The aspects of functioning and disability within the ICF, particularly body function and structure, again find a relationship with the physical component section of the Canadian Model. There is a closer relationship between the two when it comes to the Activities and Participation section of the ICF and the Canadian Model. The ICF's categories cover learning, communication, mobility, self-care, domestic life, social activities, civic and community life, all of which are incorporated by the performance areas of Self-care, Productivity and Leisure within the Canadian Model.

There is also within the contextual factors of the ICF, which include technology, the natural environment, the social environment and service environment, the same spread of potential environmental influences on the person's functioning that are present in the Canadian Model. And the area of attitudes observable as a result of customs, practices, values, norms and religious beliefs, finds itself a link not only to the aspects of culture covered in the Environment section of the Model, but also the area of Spirituality which is at the heart of the latter. As the author of Chapter 2 has acknowledged, there are some personal factors, such as age, gender, coping styles and previous experience, that are not covered by the ICF but would be in the Canadian Model, particularly in using sections of the occupational therapy process model, already discussed above, that take into account the uniqueness of the individual and therefore the person's strengths and needs and coping strategies (stage 4).

As with the Canadian Model, the ICF is designed as a conceptual framework rather than a process. As with the occupational therapy process model, which actions the Canadian Model into a working document, the same needs to happen with the ICF in terms of its application to a person, as illustrated in Chapter 2 of this book.

Seeing Shelly from the perspective of the ICF again expands from the case study into how a person could be seen from a perspective of how she functions, how the environment impacts on her and her social relationships.

One of the fundamental areas not addressed in the ICF but core to the Canadian Model is that the individual dictates what they wish to do through the use of the assessment tool of the COPM, which is the starting point of intervention. Another is the influence of the person's age on determining activities, with the Canadian Model being quite explicit about the individual's activities changing over their lifespan and therefore any COPM assessment needs to be reviewed regularly to ensure that it is current to the person's wishes.

CONCLUSION

This chapter has considered the use of the Canadian Model in relation to rehabilitation and interprofessional working. There is some research to show that occupational therapists are finding that the use of the Canadian Model and the Performance Measure give them a clearer sense of their role within the interdisciplinary team, as already has been mentioned above (Wressle et al 2003). However there has been little research into the use of the Canadian Model as a rehabilitation tool that the whole team may use, so some of the questions for practice might include:

QUESTIONS FOR PRACTICE

- Is the Canadian Model a useful model to use within an interdisciplinary team?
- What would be the disadvantages and advantages for the interdisciplinary team in using the COPM as an assessment tool?
- Where does the Canadian Model fit in the area of rehabilitation?
- What is fundamental about the model that fits it to the rehabilitation setting and where do other occupational therapy models fit in this particular environment?

References

Bodiam C 1999 The use of the Canadian Occupational Performance Measure for the assessment of outcome on a neurorehabilitation unit. British Journal of Occupational Therapy 62:123–126

Bosch J 1995 The reliability and validity of the COPM. MSc thesis, McMaster University, Montreal, Canada

Canadian Association of Occupational Therapists 1983 Guidelines for the client-centred practice of occupational therapy. CAOT, Ottawa

Chapparo C, Ranka J 1997 Occupational performance model (Australia). Monograph 1. Co-ordinates Publications, Victoria, Australia

Christiansen C 1999 The Eleanor Clark Slagle Lecture: defining lives, occupation as identity; and essay on competence, coherence and the creation of meaning. American Journal of occupational therapy 53:547–548

Christiansen C, Baum C (eds) 1997 Occupational therapy: enabling function and well-being, 2nd ed. Slack, Thorofare, NJ

Clarke C 2003 Clinical application of the Canadian Model of Occupational Performance in a forensic rehabilitation hostel. British Journal of Occupational Therapy 66:171–174

Creek J 2002 Occupational therapy and mental health, 3rd edn. Churchill Livingstone, Edinburgh

Csikszentmihalyi M 1992 Flow: the psychology of happiness. Rider, London

Digby A 1985 Moral treatment at the Retreat 1796–1846. In: Bynum W, Porter R, Shepherd M (eds) The anatomy of madness: essays on the history of psychiatry. Tavistock, London

Fearing VG 1993 Occupational therapists chart a course through the health record. Canadian Journal of Occupational Therapy 60:232–240

Fearing VG, Law M, Clark M 1997 An occupational performance process model: fostering client and therapist alliances. Canadian Journal of Occupational Therapy 64:7–15

Fedden T, Green A, Hill T 1999 Out of the woods: the Canadian Occupational Performance Measure, from the manual into practice. British Journal of Occupational Therapy 62:318–320

Fleming M 1991 The therapist with the three-track mind. American Journal of Occupational Therapy 45:1008

Frankl V 1992 Man's search for meaning: an introduction to logotherapy, 4th edn. Beacon, Boston

Gilbertson L, Langhorne P 2000 Home-based occupational therapy: stroke patients' satisfaction with occupational performance and service provision. British Journal of Occupational Therapy 63: 464–468

Hagedorn R 2000 Tools for practice in occupational therapy. Churchill Livingstone, Edinburgh

Hagedorn R 2002 Foundations for practice in occupational therapy. Churchill Livingstone, Edinburgh

Healy H, Rigby P 1999 Promoting independence for teens and young adults with physical disabilities. Canadian Journal of Occupational Therapy 66:240–259

Kelly G 1955 Psychology of personal contructs. Norton, New York

Kielhofner G 2002 Model of human occupation, 3rd ed. Lippincott Williams & Wilkins, Baltimore

Law M, Baptiste S, Carswell A et al 1990 The Canadian occupational performance measure: an outcome measure for occupational therapy. Canadian Journal of Occupational Therapy 57:82–87

Law M, Baptiste S, Carswell A et al 1994a Canadian Occupational Performance Measure. CAOT, Toronto

Law M, Baptiste S, Carswell A et al 1994b Pilot testing of the Canadian Occupational Performance Measure: clinical and measurement issues. Canadian Journal of Occupational Therapy 61:191–197

Law M, Baptiste S, Mills J 1995 Client-centred practice: what does it mean and does it make a difference? Canadian Journal of Occupational Therapy 62:250–257

Maslow A, Abraham H 1987 Motivation and personality, 3rd edn. Harper & Row, London

McColl MA, Paterson M, Davies D, Doubt L, Law M 2000 Validity and community utility of the Canadian Occupational Performance Measure. Canadian Journal of Occupational Therapy 67:22–30

Mew M, Fossey E 1996 Client-centred aspects of clinical reasoning during an initial assessment using the Canadian Occupational Performance Measure. Australian Occupational Therapy Journal 43:155–166

Morse JM, Johnson JL 1991 The illness experience: dimensions of suffering. Sage, Newbury Park, CA

Norris A 1999 A pilot study of an outcome measure in palliative care. International Journal of Palliative Nursing 5:40–45

Orem D 1985 Nursing – concepts and practice, 3rd edn. Prentice-Hall, London

Payne VG, Isaacs LD 1991 Human motor development: a lifespan approach, 2nd edn. Mayfield Publishing, Mountain View, CA

Pedretti LW, Early MB 2001 Occupational therapy: practice skills for physical dysfunction. Mosby, St Louis

Peloquin S 1991a Occupational therapy service: individual and collective understandings of the founders. American Journal of Occupational Therapy 45:352 260

Peloquin S 1991b Occupational therapy service: individual and collective understandings of the founders. American Journal of Occupational Therapy 45:733–744

Polatajko H 1992 Naming and framing occupational therapy: a lecture dedicated to the memory of Nancy B. Canadian Journal of Occupational therapy 59:189–200

Pollock N 1993 Client-centred assessment. American Journal of Occupational Therapy 47:298–301

Reed KL, Sanderson SN 1984 Models of practice in occupational therapy. Wilkins & Wilkins, Baltimore

Reed KL, Sanderson SN 1992 Concepts of occupational therapy 3rd edn. Wilkins & Wilkins, Baltimore

Rogers C 1986 On becoming a person. Constable, London

Roper N, Logan W, Tierney A 1990 The elements of nursing. Churchill Livingstone, Edinburgh

Roy C 1984 An introduction to nursing: an adaptation model, 2nd edn. Prentice Hall, Englewood Cliffs, NJ

Schkade J, Schultz S 1997 Occupational adaptation model. In: Christiansen C, Sewell L, Singh S 2001 The Canadian Occupational Performance Measure: is it a reliable measure in clients with Chronic obstructive pulmonary disease? British Journal of Occupational Therapy 54:386–392

Stewart A 1992 The Casson Memorial lecture: always a little further. British Journal of Occupational Therapy 54:297–300

Sumsion T (ed) 1999 Client-centred practice in occupational therapy. Churchill Livingstone, Edinburgh

Toomey M. Nicholson D, Carswell A 1995 The clinical utility of the Canadian Occupational Performance Measure. Canadian Journal of Occupational Therapy 62:242–249

Townsend E (ed) 1997 Enabling occupation: an occupational therapy perspective. Canadian Association of Occupational Therapy, Ottawa

Townsend E, Brintnell S, Staisey N 1990 Developing guidelines for client-centred occupational therapy practice. Canadian Journal of Occupational Therapy 57:69–76

Trombly CA, Vining Radomski M, Davis ES 1998 Achievement of self-identified goals by adults with traumatic brain injury: phase 1. American Journal of Occupational Therapy 52:810–818

Tryssenaar J, Jones E, Lee D 1999 Occupational performance needs of a shelter population. Canadian Journal of Occupational Therapy 66:188–196

Wade DT, de Jong BA 2000 Recent advances in rehabilitation. British Medical Journal 320:1385–1388

Waters D 1995 Recovering from a depressive episode using the Canadian Occupational Performance Measure. Canadian Journal of Occupational Therapy 62:278–282.

Whiteneck CG 1994 Measuring what matters: key rehabilitation outcomes. Archives of Physical Medicine and Rehabilitation 75:1073–1076

World Health Organization 2001 International classification of Functioning and Disability. World Health Organization, Geneva

Wilcock A 1998 An occupational perspective of health. Slack, Thorofare, NJ.

Wressle E, Eeg-Olofsson AM; Marcusson J, Henriksson C 2002 Improved client participation in the rehabilitation process using an client-centred goal formulation structure. Journal of Rehabilitation and Medicine 34:5–11

Wressle E, Lindstrand, J, Neher, M, Marcusson J, Henriksson C 2003 The Canadian occupational performance measure as an outcome measure and team tool in a day treatment programme. Disability and Rehabilitation 25:497–506

Wressle E, Samuelsson K, Henriksson C 1999 Responsiveness of the Swedish version of the Canadian Occupational Performance Measure. Scandinavian Journal of Occupational Therapy 6:84–89

Wright J. 2004 Occupation and flow. In: Molineux M. Occupation for occupational therapists. Blackwell, Oxford, p 66–77

Yerxa EJ, Clark F, Frank G, Jackson J, Parham D, Pierce D, Stein C, Zemke R. 1989 An introduction to occupational science: a foundation for occupational therapy in the twenty-first century. Occupational Therapy in Health Care 6:1–17

Zemke R, Clark F (eds) 1996 Occupational science: the evolving discipline FA Davis,. Philadelphia

Chapter **5**

The Illness Constellation Model

Sally Davis

INTRODUCTION

Rehabilitation is a complex process because there are different variables that contribute to it. One of these is what the experience means for that individual. How are they dealing with their illness? It doesn't matter whether the illness is a long-term chronic condition or more acute. It may also be classified as trauma rather than illness. In order for health-care professionals to respond appropriately it is important for them to understand how different individuals might see and deal with their illness. One model that helps understand this experience is the Illness Constellation Model, which was developed, by Morse & Johnson (1991) in response to the need for a more comprehensive framework that might help to explain how individuals view illness and behave towards it. The aim of this chapter is to:

- Describe the model and its development
- Explore its relationship to rehabilitation and the implications for interprofessional working
- Discuss it in relationship to other models
- Discuss it in relationship to the International Classification of Functioning and Health
- Relate the model to case studies.

THE MODEL

Morse & Johnson (1991) developed the Illness Constellation Model using five grounded theory studies, which looked at the experience of chronic illness for different individuals. These studies covered the experience of:

- Adjusting to a heart attack
- Women having a hysterectomy
- Individuals with schizophrenia leaving the psychiatric hospital
- Mothers' involvement in their adolescent
- Husbands during their wives' chemotherapy.

Although these are very different experiences of illness Morse & Johnson (1991) were able to identify similarities between the stages that individuals go through during their experience of chronic illness. The studies focused very much on what the experience of chronic illness was like for that individual and their significant others.

Morse & Johnson (1991) point out that illness is generally conceptualised in terms of the individual's experience of symptoms, which is synonymous with the medical model, or in terms of their ability to cope with the illness, which can be identified as an adaptation or coping model. Both these views of illness are limited and take no real account of the actual experience of being ill, for the individual and their significant others. In practice the relationships between the individual undergoing rehabilitation and their family undergo many phases, in which at times either the individual or the family is compensating in response to the illness/incident. The individual goes through stages of feeling ill and wanting to relinquish control to the realisation that things may not improve and that they need to begin to accept this and internalise it to enable them to get on with their life.

The Illness Constellation Model (Morse & Johnson 1991) identifies this and describes four main stages that the individual and others go through (Table 5.1). The first two stages of uncertainty and disruption are characterised by the individual losing control, whereas stages 3 and 4 are about the individual regaining control. For 'relevant others' this progression is almost reversed, with the first two stages being where they are perhaps taking more control and then relinquishing that in stages 3 and 4.

It is useful to consider the stages in relation to the Trajectory of Illness Framework identified by Corbin & Strauss (1991), which describes the experience of chronic illness. The Trajectory of Illness Framework was developed using a grounded theory approach looking at the experience of dying. It has been applied to different types of chronic illness: cardiac illness (Hawthorne 1991), cancer (Dorsett 1992), multiple sclerosis (Miller 1993), diabetes (Walker 1992) and stroke rehabilitation (Burton 2000). It has also been used to look at elderly patients with chronic illness (Robinson et al 1993). The Trajectory of Illness framework consists of eight stages: pre-trajectory, trajectory, crisis, acute, stable, unstable, downward and dying. Table 5.2 shows a comparison of these stages with the stages in the Illness Constellation Model.

One of the things the Trajectory of Illness Framework makes explicit, which the Illness Constellation Model does not, is that the phases may not all be positive. It takes into account that challenges individuals may face may cause them to deteriorate. It implies more of a cyclical ongoing process, whereas the Illness Constellation Model identifies stages an individual will go through. The Illness Constellation Model implies that there is an end; however, for some individuals this end may not be reached. This view is supported by Jarrett (2000) who identified a model of coping that highlights the transitional process of living with a chronic illness. Jarrett's model incorporates elements of the Illness Constellation Model and elements of the Trajectory of Illness Framework and makes explicit the fact that adaptation, adjustment and mastery are not

Table 5.1   The stages of the Illness Constellation Model

Stage	Self/Sick Person	Significant Others
1. Uncertainty	*Suspecting*: Signs of illness; feeling unwell/unsettled	*Suspecting*: Becoming aware something serious is happening
	Reading the body: Is this normal?	*Monitoring*: for symptoms
	Being overwhelmed: physically and emotionally	*Becoming overwhelmed*: by worry and concern; the illness is a reality
2. Disruption	*Relinquishing control*: Choices and decisions are made by others	*Accepting responsibility*: They feel a need to help in any way
	Distancing oneself: Things seem unreal	*Being vigilant*: Waiting to see if they are needed
3. Striving to regain self	*Making sense*: Coming to terms with what the illness means	*Committed to the struggle*: Using all their efforts
	Preserving self: Begin to assert themselves to reclaim control	*Buffering*: Protecting the individual from worry and concern
	Renegotiating roles and responsibilities: Accepting and relinquishing	*Renegotiating roles and responsibilities*: Accepting and relinquishing
	Setting goals: in order to feel they are making progress	*Monitoring activities*: to ensure that the individual isn't overdoing it
	Seeking reassurance: to help that sense of uncertainty	*Supporting*: giving praise and encouragement
4. Regaining wellness	*Taking charge*: Relationships gradually return to resemble former patterns	*Making it through*: Continue to be concerned about the future
	Seeking closure: Resolving what has happened to them	*Seeking closure*: Putting the illness behind them

Source: With permission from Morse & Johnson 1991.

definitive endpoints in the process of chronic illness. They are ways in which individuals move in the transition process and do not have to be achieved in order for an individual to be considered well.

The Illness Constellation Model can be considered in terms of a cyclical process where individuals may move through each stage, may remain in one stage or may go back through the stages. An individual may remain in stage 3 but feel they have adapted to their illness. It could be said that the Illness Constellation Model is more of a model of wellness than illness, with stage 4 being focused on regaining wellness.

Table 5.2 Comparison of the stage of the Trajectory of Illness Framework and the Illness Constellation Model

Trajectory of Illness Framework	Illness Constellation Model
Pre-trajectory: Occurs before the onset of symptoms	Stage 1: Where the individual is suspecting that something is wrong
Trajectory onset: Signs and symptoms appear	Signs and symptoms would appear in Stage 2
Crisis phase: The signs and symptoms pose a threat to the individual's physical, social or psychological integrity	Stage 2: Where the individual is experiencing disruption and relinquishing control
Acute phase: Active intervention is required	Active intervention could occur at Stages 2 and 3; in Stages 3 and 4 the individual is beginning to take control
Stable phase: Intervention is effective and a period of stability has been reached	Stage 3: The individual is making sense of what is happening – this could be seen as a period of stability
Unstable phase: The individual may experience challenges to their recovery, which may require them to reappraise the situation	Stage 3: The individual may need to renegotiate roles and responsibilities and set and renegotiate goals; if the individual is unable to respond to the challenges they may go back to stage 2
Downward phase: The individual is not able to respond to the challenges and their condition may deteriorate	Stage 2: The individual will go back to the disruption stage where they are relinquishing control
Dying: the time leading up to death	This is not explicitly mentioned in the Illness Constellation Model. It could be associated with Stage 2; however, at this point the individual may feel at peace with themselves and feel they are seeking closure, as identified in *stage 4*. This may be the same for significant others

REHABILITATION

The Illness Constellation Model fits in with the aims of rehabilitation, which can be seen as maximising an individual's quality of life and focusing on wellness. This fits in with the Health Promotion Model (Davis 1995) discussed in Chapter 2, which highlights the link between rehabilitation and health promotion, the focus of both being on wellness. The Illness Constellation Model, with its focus on control, fits in with the notion of autonomy for the individual that is highlighted in the Kings Fund definition of rehabilitation (Sinclair & Dickinson 1998), which describes rehabilitation as a process aimed at restoring personal autonomy. One way for individuals to regain personal autonomy is for them to set their own goals, which is the focus of stage 3 of the Illness Constellation Model. The stages of rehabilitation as identified in Chapter 1 can be linked to the Illness Constellation Model (Table 5.3).

Table 5.3 Stages of rehabilitation and the stages in the Illness Constellation Model

Stage of Rehabilitation	Stage in the Illness Constellation Model
Stage 1: Initial critical stage – goal is to maintain life	*Stage 2*: The individual is relinquishing control and depending on health-care professionals
Stage 2: Regaining some physical function – goal will depend on needs; maybe to maintain a safe, comfortable environment	*Stage 3*: The individual is beginning to make sense of what is happening; maybe focusing on regaining some physical function
Stage 3: More active programme of rehabilitation – goal is concerned with the individual's quality of life	*Stage 3*: The individual is renegotiating roles and responsibilities and setting goals, taking a much more active role
Stage 4: Individual reached full potential – focus is on them living with their disabilities and maintaining their quality of life	*Stage 4*: The individual is feeling confident with their abilities, relationships are returning to their former state, they are able to seek some closure

In terms of rehabilitation it is useful to consider each stage of the Illness Constellation Model and to discuss the related concepts. Each stage will be related to the stories of Chan and Myrtle, the case studies detailed in Chapter 2. An issue to consider that is particularly pertinent in rehabilitation where there is a close relationship with the team is that 'others' could be considered as being the multi or interdisciplinary team.

Stage 1: Uncertainty

At this stage the individual is beginning to suspect something is wrong but may not be able to identify what it is. Their family may be suspecting that something is not right and may be extremely concerned and worried. Rehabilitation would probably not begin at this stage, as the individual may not be in the health-care system. However, health promotion is an important aspect to consider at this stage as it can prepare individuals to recognise the signs that something may be wrong. For example having read leaflets on breast examination and consequently carrying it out would then enable a woman to read the signs that something is not right. In order for individuals to know what is 'normal' with regards to their body they may need education and knowledge. This may come in the form of leaflets, media, discussion with others, journals and books.

CASE STUDY CHAN

Chan (42, had a stroke) did not feel right in himself before the stroke. He felt generally unwell. Chan had been given advice about his high blood pressure but did not follow it. He did know that he was at risk of having a stroke. Chan's wife had been worried for some time about Chan's blood pressure and had been urging him to follow the doctor's advice. Although Chan had not been his usual self, she had put it down to overwork and tiredness. Chan's children had sensed that something wasn't right with their dad and tended to avoid him.

Myrtle (75, fractured left neck of femur) did not have any idea that this was about to happen. Myrtle had become more anxious since fracturing her right neck of femur and was worried about the number of falls she had had. This was also a concern for her family, in particular Cassie (her eldest daughter, who visited often and was close to her mother), who had repeatedly tried to get Myrtle to wear her spectacles. The staff in the nursing home had also been concerned at Myrtle's poor eyesight and lapses of concentration. They had tried where possible to ensure that Myrtle was not left alone.

Stage 2: Disruption

At this stage the individual has become ill and needs to relinquish control to others, which will more than likely be health-care professionals. For the individual things may seem unreal and there may be a sense that things are happening to someone else. Significant others may want to help in any way they can so that they don't feel useless. Morse & Johnson (1991) and McGonigal (1998) identify stages 3 and 4 as being stages of rehabilitation. However, if rehabilitation is to be thought of as beginning from the moment of onset of illness or trauma, then this would include stage 2, as shown in Table 5.3.

Paterson & Stewart (2002) conducted a small study to describe how adults with traumatic brain injury perceived their social interactions and relationships. Three categories were identified: diminished concentration, disrupted feelings and emotions, and redefining self. Although only a small sample of six participants was used the results support the levels of the Illness Constellation Model. In the category of disrupted feelings and emotions, participants described changes in feelings and emotions that were a result of having reduced control over anger and frustration. This was accompanied by loss of motivation. This category supports stage 2 of the Illness Constellation Model, where individuals feel that they have no control and that their life has been disrupted.

At this stage, Chan was semiconscious for a few days; he was unable to communicate and relied on health-care professionals to take control. When Chan regained consciousness he still required a lot of help and felt out of control. Health-care professionals took control to ensure that Chan was not in any danger and to prevent complications. Chan's wife wanted to look after Chan at this stage and spent a lot of time by his side. She felt frustrated that she wasn't able to care for him fully. The health-care professionals supported her at this stage by giving her information and talking through what was happening to Chan. They also put her in touch with the Stroke Association, who were able to put her in touch with someone locally whose husband had also had a stroke.

CASE STUDY MYRTLE

Immediately following her fall, Myrtle was in a lot of pain and was happy for the doctors to take control. She quickly had a hip operation and was quite unwell for a few days following it. The team took control at this stage and their focus was to ensure that Myrtle did not suffer from any complications and that she had adequate pain control. Myrtle's eldest daughter, Cassie, was able to visit Myrtle every day. The rest of Myrtle's family were not able to visit but they rang regularly. Cassie felt that at times the nurses in the ward did not take much notice of Myrtle. This feeling resulted in Cassie being angry with the nurses. One of the reasons for this feeling was that Cassie felt helpless at not being able to do anything for her mother and felt guilty that Myrtle had fallen. She had been trying unsuccessfully to get Myrtle to wear her spectacles and felt that if she had succeeded Myrtle would not have fallen. She also felt that her brothers and sisters blamed her for Myrtle's fall. Cassie was unable to share these feelings with the health-care professionals. At this stage Cassie might have benefited from one-to-one support from a member of the team.

Stage 3: Striving to regain self

At this stage the individual is beginning to come to terms with the consequences of the illness or disability. There is a need at this stage for individuals to begin to take back some control, which can affect their own self-concept and confidence. The second category of Paterson & Stewart's study (2002) was 'redefining of self': participants described how perceptions of themselves as individuals had been affected by changes in their social interactions and relationships with family and friends. This category fits in with stage 3, in which the individual is striving to make sense of what is happening and is renegotiating roles. Fundamental to rehabilitation is the need for individuals to set their own goals and to participate as fully as possible in their care. This means that individuals need to have some control over the rehabilitation process. In stage 3 individuals are beginning to take back this control. Burks (1999), in the development of a nursing practice model for chronic illness, identifies self-management as being a key concept in relation to rehabilitation. This is in terms of the individual's role in decision-making and goal setting.

Developing a sense of self can also be seen as a spiritual journey (Nosek & Hughes 2001). Self is related to self-concept and self-esteem. In terms of 'others' in the Illness Constellation Model, therapeutic use of self is important to health-care practitioners, who use themselves in a therapeutic way. Pizzi & Briggs (2004) identify the importance of health-care practitioners developing an awareness of themselves. This means health-care practitioners seeing the personal consequences of illness for the individual, responding to individuals in an understanding and empathetic way and establishing a two-way relationship. This view is supported by Hwu (1995) in a study exploring the impact of chronic illness on 177 patients in China. The study concluded that it is important for health-care professionals to understand the experience of chronic illness for the individual and to understand how individuals respond to it. The need for a holistic assessment, discharge planning and follow-up of patients was highlighted.

CASE STUDY CHAN

Chan has been making sense of what it will mean to him to have had a stroke. He has been speaking to members of the rehabilitation team about the consequences of his stroke. Chan has been feeling angry at what has happened to him and has found it difficult to come to terms with the stroke. Chan has lost confidence in his abilities but has begun to identify goals with the team. He has not been able to discuss issues with his wife: he feels he will lose face with his wife and the community if he cannot resume his role as a husband and father. At this stage Chan is facing a number of challenges, which he is finding difficult to deal with. He could progress on to stage 4 or he could go back to stage 2. The support he gets at this point is essential.

Chan's wife is trying to protect Chan as much as possible from the challenges that have arisen as a result of his stroke. These challenges include the possibility of Chan not returning to work, not being able to drive and the home environment being unsuitable. The relationship between Chan and his wife since the stroke has been strained, which has been difficult for them both as one of their strengths as a couple was that they supported each other, discussed everything and made decisions together. For Chan this loss has felt like a bereavement. He doesn't believe that his wife feels the same as before, when in fact she does. For Chan to get through this stage he and his wife need to resume their relationship, both physically and psychologically. The team could help facilitate this by helping Chan and his wife identify goals towards this. This may include Chan and his wife spending some time together and maybe having time at home.

CASE STUDY MYRTLE

Myrtle has not wanted to take control: she has been happy for the doctors and health-care professionals to make decisions for her. This fits in with Myrtle's behaviour since living in the nursing home, where she has mainly had an external locus of control, particularly where professionals are concerned. She has always felt happy to relinquish control and follow instructions. The team have tried to enable her to identify goals that are important to her. Myrtle's family have regular discussions about Myrtle and feel that the team should be pushing Myrtle towards being independent in aspects of physical care. Cassie, as the spokesperson for the family, has had talks with the team about this. The team have identified how Myrtle is and feel that encouraging her too much would result in her not wanting to do anything but lie in bed. They are therefore identifying small goals for Myrtle to achieve. They have tried to explain this to Cassie but Cassie believes they should be doing more and has the attitude that they need to be cruel to be kind.

Myrtle is really still in stage 2, whereas her family and the health-care professionals are at stage 3. In terms of self, Myrtle has gained a lot of her strength from the Church. This is the same for her family, who all hold deeply religious beliefs. To some degree Myrtle feels that God will look after her. Cassie, although believing strongly in God, realises that Myrtle needs to make some effort if she is to regain some independence and control.

| Stage 4: Regaining wellness | At this stage the individual is beginning to take charge of their life to regain wellness. Wellness in the literature is described as encompassing spirituality, physical health, social engagement and environment. Wellness can be considered to be a multilevel phenomenon that encompasses the person, the community and the social and physical environment (Putnam et al 2003). Putnam et al (2003) conducted a study to explore how people living with long-term disabilities conceptualise health and |

wellness. 99 adults between the ages of 22 and 82 were included in the study, with long-term disabilities including multiple sclerosis, cerebral palsy and spinal cord injury. The participants identified the following characteristics of health and wellness:

- Being able to function at a level that enables them to do what they want to do
- Being self-determining or independent
- Having an emotional state of wellbeing as well as physical wellbeing
- Having no pain.

For the majority of participants being able to perform necessary or desired daily activities was an important measure of health and wellness.

As a result of the study Putnam et al (2003) identified that interventions to promote health and wellness could take place at different levels:

- *Individual level*: the development of coping strategies, interacting with peer groups, staying active, contributing to society, setting personal goals and challenges
- *Community level*: interacting socially with friends and family, feeling valued by friends and family and others in the community
- *Health-care professionals*: being respectful and informed and concerned with the total person
- *Systems level*: accessible environment and accessible accommodation.

Mastery is a feature of stage 4. Morse & Johnson (1991) talk about it as individuals trusting their abilities. It is about being in control and having skills. It can be seen as being related to self-efficacy, identified by Bandura (1997) as being the ability of individuals to adapt to a stressful situation as illness or a new disability by reorganising cognitive, social and behavioural skills to adapt to the situation. Hampton (2004), in a study of 127 participants exploring wellbeing among people with spinal cord injuries, found that there was a strong correlation between self-efficacy and perceived social support to subjective wellbeing. The study concluded that, in order to increase an individual's wellbeing, rehabilitation must incorporate training programmes that enhance self-efficacy and social support. Self-efficacy was found to be related to an individual's level of confidence. Airlie et al (2001) developed a self-efficacy scale for people with multiple sclerosis. The scale which can be used by professionals to measure an individual's level of self-efficacy, covers questions on the amount of control individuals feel they have and what affects that control. It also focuses on the way individuals cope.

CASE STUDY CHAN

Chan is now at home with his family. He has adapted to his situation to a degree. He has learned new skills to enable him to be independent and he is able to negotiate the stairs in his house. He has been given some equipment to enable him to bath independently. With the support of a clinical psychologist, Chan and his wife have begun to talk about the implications of the stroke. They are still both seeing the psychologist on an outpatient basis. While in the unit they were also able to talk to a nurse about the sexual side of their relationship. She was able to give them some written information and talk this through with them. As a result of this support Chan has felt more confident and feels he is beginning to resume his role as a husband. There are still issues around Chan returning to work, which are a result of his employers' views. Chan wants to return to work; this is to him an important element of him as a man. The community occupational therapist is discussing the issues with Chan's employers and it looks as if they will find a part-time role for him. Chan and his wife have been supported by their neighbours and friends. There is a strong sense of community where they live. It could be said that Chan has developed self-efficacy by reorganising his skills and behaviour to adapt to the situation.

CASE STUDY MYRTLE

Myrtle is now back in the nursing home. She has recovered from her hip operation and is functioning physically as she was before the fall; however, she is much more anxious and constantly calls for the nurses. There are still issues with her not wearing her spectacles and being forgetful. Myrtle has maybe accepted that this is a normal state for her and feels that in terms of control she has as much as she wants. It could be argued whether Myrtle is at stage 4 in terms of regaining mastery. Perhaps she has regained wellness in terms of being at the level she was before. It could be said that Myrtle has almost skipped stage 3, as she only regained a limited amount of control, which could be seen as her way of coping with events. This would fit in with Myrtle's previous coping style. Cassie has resumed her routine of visiting Myrtle three or four times a week in the nursing home. Cassie feels she has a huge weight on her shoulders as she is constantly in fear of Myrtle falling again. She feels she is not able to relinquish control, so remains at stage 3, in which she tries to protect Myrtle and monitors what Myrtle is doing. The rest of Myrtle's family are in constant contact with Cassie about Myrtle, which is stressful for Cassie. Cassie is not able to seek any kind of closure to the event.

LOCUS OF CONTROL

As control is a feature of the Illness Constellation Model it is useful to consider the concept of locus of control. The relevance of this is highlighted in the story of Myrtle. The theory of locus of control (King 1984) refers to how much an individual thinks their actions affect events that happen generally to them. Two main types of locus of control are identified:

- *Internal locus*: Individuals believe that they are able to make a difference and that they have control over what happens to them
- *External locus*: Individuals believe that others control their lives and that they are unable to make a difference.

There is little research on the implications of locus of control for rehabilitation and the effect it may have on rehabilitation outcomes. Norman & Norman (1991) looked at the relationship of individuals' health locus of control beliefs to progress in rehabilitation and found that participants who believed in internal locus of control progressed in rehabilitation more than those who believed in external locus of control. There were 93 participants in the study but it is not explicit what their chronic illness or disability was. Younger et al (1995) looked at the relationship between locus of control and cardiac rehabilitation to mastery of illness-related stress. The sample consisted of 111 individuals who were in hospital with coronary artery disease. The results showed some correlation of internal locus of control to growth and total mastery and some correlation to change.

It could be said that individuals generally tend to be more of one type than the other; however, we all dip in and out of internal and external locus depending on events that happen to us. In terms of chronic illness and disability an individual with a generally internal locus may take on an external locus, thereby relinquishing control when they are acutely ill – in relation to the Illness Constellation Model, in stage 2. It is important for professionals to recognise where individuals are in terms of their locus of control as this can have an effect on how they adapt to their illness. This is evident with Myrtle, where the team are working in accordance with her locus of control and by doing that they are able to help Myrtle to achieve some small goals. Applying the Illness Constellation Model, someone with a mostly internal locus may go through the stages more quickly than someone with an external locus. Someone with an external locus may not achieve level 4, where the focus is on taking charge and attaining mastery. This point of view is supported by Younger et al (1995). This focus on control is emphasised in the National Service Frameworks for older people (Department of Health 2001) and the forthcoming National Service Framework on long-term conditions. In order for individuals to regain control, rehabilitation professionals need to move away from thinking in terms of the disease process – a feature of the medical model (Morse & Johnson 1991) – to more of a problem solving approach in terms of the individual and their environment.

Rehabilitation professionals need to rethink strategies that enable individuals to question their own potential and take responsibility for improving their own health (McGonigal 1998). However, it is important that these strategies take into account an individual's locus of control. Table 5.4 relates rehabilitation strategies to the levels of the Illness Constellation Model.

COPING

The Illness Constellation Model is really about the way individuals adapt to and cope with their changed circumstances. The way people adapt and cope depends on how they see the situation and the resources they have to cope with and adapt to it. Coping is the process individuals go through to manage external or internal demands that they identify as being too much for them to resolve. They feel they do not have the physical or psychological resources (Lazarus & Folkman 1984). In their model of coping, Lazarus & Folkman (1984) identify that individuals appraise the situation in the following ways:

- *Primary appraisal*: The stressor is appraised in terms of the harm or loss it may cause and in terms of future threats and the degree of challenge it causes. For example, Chan saw the stroke as affecting his

Table 5.4 Stages of the Illness Constellation Model and rehabilitation strategies

Stage of Illness Constellation Model	Goal of Rehabilitation	Strategies
Stage 1: Uncertainty	Prevention of illness	Displaying and providing information
	Raising people's awareness	Screening for potential problems (e.g. blood pressure, glucose monitoring) and abnormalities
Stage 2: Disruption	Prevention of complications	Monitoring individual's physical state
	Maintaining life and safe environment	Supporting significant others Supporting the individual
Stage 3: Striving to	For individual to take control regain self	Assessment of individual's strengths, weaknesses, health beliefs Setting realistic goals Promoting empowerment Assessment of environment Focus on relationships
Stage 4: Regaining wellness	For individuals to remain at their optimum state of wellness	Support in the community Assertiveness training Counselling Financial support Monitoring access Promoting social interaction

whole life, causing him losses in terms of independence, work and in his relationship with his wife. It gave him a lot of challenges to face

● *Secondary appraisal*: The coping resources and options an individual has are appraised. Chan usually coped with events by discussing them with his wife. Chan has identified that there is a difficulty with his relationship with his wife, which has affected the way he copes.

These levels of appraisal relate to stage 3 of the Illness Constellation Model.

Other elements identified by Lazarus & Folkman (1984) that relate to the model are:

● *Coping responses and strategies*: Information seeking, direct action, turning to others. For Chan and his wife this involves seeking information and receiving support from the team in particular the clinical psychologist

● *Coping tasks*: Reducing harmful environmental conditions, maintaining a positive self-image, continuing satisfying relationships. Chan was able to achieve a positive self-image by identifying and achieving goals and seeking support. He and his wife also worked at resuming their relationship. Having some adaptations to his home also helped him cope with the situation

● *Coping outcomes*: Psychological outcomes, resuming usual activities, physiological changes. Chan achieved outcomes in terms of his psychological and emotional state. He was able to resume most of his usual activities. In terms of physiological changes he achieved a level of physical independence.

Other factors that affect the way an individual copes are their personality, other life stressors, social support, money, time and usual coping styles (Lazarus & Folkman 1984). For Chan there were issues around money. When discharged home he had a lot of social support in terms of family, friends and neighbours.

RELATIONSHIP TO THE INTERNATIONAL CLASSIFICATION OF FUNCTIONING, DISABILITY AND HEALTH

In terms of the ICF the Illness Constellation Model relates mostly to Part 1: Functioning and Disability and Part 2: Contextual Factors. The changes an individual has in terms of their body functions and structures will affect the way they perform in activities, which in turn may affect the way they deal with the situation. For example, the loss of function in Chan's left arm and leg has decreased his level of independence, which he has found difficult to deal with. At stage 3 this has caused him challenges, which have prevented him moving on to stage 4 at a quicker pace. One of the issues the ICF emphasises that could affect the stages people go through in the Illness Constellation Model is the difference there may be between the capacity an individual has in terms of activities and their actual performance. For example, Myrtle does have the capacity to wash and dress herself but she continually asks for assistance. She has taken on a role of dependence rather than independence. This would suggest that there are issues in terms of control for Myrtle, which may account for the difficulty in her moving through stage 3 and on to stage 4.

Environmental factors, as identified in the ICF, may also have an effect on the stages of the Illness Constellation Model. There may be external influences that will affect the way an individual deals with their illness and how they move through the stages in the Illness Constellation Model. For example, there is an issue for Chan in terms of his employers' attitude towards him returning to work. This could be a difficult challenge for him to cope with and as a result he could revert back to stage 2, in which he wants others to make decisions for him. In the early stages of his stroke Chan wasn't able to return to his house because of the access difficulties due to the steps. This factor may have hindered his progression from stage 2 to stage 3. Within the section on environmental factors in the ICF is a chapter on support and relationships.

Perhaps one of the most important areas that the ICF can help with in terms of individuals moving through the stages of the Illness Constellation Model is in the recognition of personal factors. How an individual deals with their illness or disability is perhaps dependent mostly on them as a person, on the type of personality they have. In the ICF, personal factors are described as the particular background of the individual and may include gender, race, age, lifestyle, coping styles, character, etc. The way both Chan and Myrtle deal with their illness is influenced by personal factors: being Chinese, Chan's culture makes it difficult for him to accept the change of role that might occur as a result of his stroke. Myrtle has always been a determined woman and can be quite obstinate about things. This side of her personality occasionally comes through when she becomes determined that she won't do as rehabilitation professionals ask. This determination and obstinacy is also evident in her daughter Cassie.

CONCLUSION

The Illness Constellation Model enables rehabilitation professionals to focus on health and wellness rather than illness. It gives professionals a framework with which to consider the illness experience for individuals and the consequences of the different stages for rehabilitation. The Illness Constellation Model considers the experience not only for individuals but also for their significant others. This category could also be used to include the health-care team. The Illness Constellation Model could be used to complement the ICF in addressing the concept of control and mastery for individuals. These are two areas that are not explicit in the ICF.

QUESTIONS FOR DISCUSSION

- What factors affect the illness experience for individuals in your practice area?
- How do the stages in the Illness Constellation Model apply to your practice area?
- What strategies do you use as a team to enable individuals to reach stage 4 of the model?

References

Airlie J, Baker GA, Smith SJ 2001 Measuring the impact of multiple sclerosis on psychosocial functioning: the development of a new self-efficacy scale. Clinical Rehabilitation 15:259–265

Bandura A 1997 Social learning theory. Prentice-Hall, Englewood Cliffs, NJ

Burks KJ 1999 A nursing practice model for chronic illness. Rehabilitation Nursing 24: 197–200

Burton CR 2000 Re-thinking stroke rehabilitation: the Corbin and Strauss chronic illness trajectory framework. Journal of Advanced Nursing 32: 595–602

Corbin JM, Strauss A 1991 A nursing model for chronic illness management based upon the trajectory framework. Scholarly Inquiry for Nursing Practice 5:155–174

Davis SM 1995 An investigation into nurses' understanding of health education and health promotion within a neuro-rehabilitation setting. Journal of Advanced Nursing 21:951–959

Department of Health 2001 National service framework for older people. HMSO, Norwich

Dorsett DS 1992 The trajectory of cancer recovery. In: Woog P (ed) The chronic illness trajectory framework. Springer, New York

Hampton NZ 2004 Subjective well-being among people with spinal cord injuries: the role of self-efficacy, perceived social support, and perceived health. Rehabilitation Counselling Bulletin 48:31–37

Hawthorne MH 1991 Using the trajectory framework: reconceptualising cardiac illness. Scholarly Inquiry for Nursing Practice 5:185–195

Hwu YJ 1995 The impact of chronic illness on patients. Rehabilitation Nursing 20:221–225

Jarrett L 2000 Living with chronic illness: a transitional model of coping. British Journal of Rehabilitation 7:40–44

King J 1984 Your health in your hands. Nursing Times 80(44):51–52

Lazarus RS, Folkman S 1984 Stress, appraisal and coping. Springer, New York

McGonigal GC 1998 Empowering health in chronic illness: a conceptual model. British Journal of Therapy and Rehabilitation 5:591–595

Miller CM 1993 Trajectory and empowerment theory applied to care of patients with multiple sclerosis. Journal of Neuroscience Nursing 25:343–348

Morse JM and Johnson JL 1991 The illness experience: dimensions of suffering. Sage Publications, Newbury Park, CA

Norman EJ, Norman VL 1991 Relationship of patient's health locus of control beliefs to progress in rehabilitation. Journal of Rehabilitation 57:27–30

Nosek MA, Hughes RB 2001 Psychospiritual aspects of sense of self in women with physical disabilities. Journal of Rehabilitation 67:20–25

Paterson J, Stewart J 2002 Adults with acquired brain injury: perceptions of their social world. Rehabilitation Nursing 27:13–18

Pizzi MA, Briggs R 2004 Occupational and physical therapy in hospice: the facilitation of meaning, quality of life and well-being. Topics in Geriatric Rehabilitation 20:120–130

Putnam M, Geenan S, Powers L 2003 Health and wellness: people with disabilities discuss barriers and facilitators to well being. Journal of Rehabilitation 69:37–45

Robinson LA, Bevil C, Arcangelo V et al 1993 Operationalising the Corbin and Strauss trajectory model for elderly clients with chronic illness. Scholarly Inquiry for Nursing Practice 7:253–268

Sinclair A, Dickinson E 1998 Effective practice in rehabilitation: evidence from systematic reviews. Kings Fund, London

Walker EA 1992 Shaping the course of a marathon: using the trajectory framework for diabetes mellitus. In Woog P (ed) The chronic illness trajectory framework. Springer, New York

World Health Organization 2001 International classification of functioning, disability and health. World Health Organization, Geneva

Younger J, Marsh KJ, Grap MJ 1995 The relationship of health locus of control and cardiac rehabilitation to mastery of illness-related stress. Journal of Advanced Nursing 22:194–299

Chapter **6**

From PLISSIT to Ex-PLISSIT

Sally Davis, Bridget Taylor

INTRODUCTION

The PLISSIT model has been used across a wide range of different client groups to consider clients' sexuality and sexual health-care needs. This chapter will explore the use of the PLISSIT model and will suggest an extended model: Ex-PLISSIT. The aims of this chapter are to:

- Consider the development of the PLISSIT model and its uses
- Explore the limitations of the PLISSIT model and describe the Ex-PLISSIT model
- Relate the Ex-PLISSIT model to the International Classification of Functioning, Disability and Health and to rehabilitation
- Apply the Ex-PLISSIT model to rehabilitation using a case study
- Share examples from practice of the use of the PLISSIT model
- Identify a training programme to prepare rehabilitation professionals in the use of the Ex-PLISSIT model.

THE PLISSIT MODEL

PLISSIT is a model that was developed by Annon (1976), an American psychosexual therapist. It was designed to assist health-care practitioners in their interventions with clients on issues of sexuality. The acronym PLISSIT signifies the four levels of intervention: Permission (P), limited information (LI), specific suggestion (SS) and intensive therapy (IT). As the level of intervention increases, greater knowledge, training and skills are required (Seidl et al 1991).

- *Level 1*: **P**ermission for the client to express concerns regarding sexuality
- *Level 2*: **L**imited **I**nformation provided
- *Level 3*: **S**pecific **S**uggestions made
- *Level 4*: **I**ntensive **T**herapy given.

According to Annon (1976), most people experiencing sexual problems can resolve them if they are given permission to be sexual, to desire sexual activity and to discuss sexuality, and if they receive limited information about sexual matters and specific suggestions about ways to address sexual problems. Annon (1976) suggests that few people need intensive therapy to resolve their sexual problems.

Practitioners are not expected to be able to function at all levels in all situations (Annon 1976). It is important that practitioners recognise their own strengths and limitations and, where necessary, refer clients on to others who are more able to address an individual client's needs. In this way, practitioners are encouraged to work within the limits of their own comfort zone and competence.

The PLISSIT model is advocated by many authors and proposed as an appropriate framework on which practitioners can base their interventions with clients. It has been recommended for use in pregnancy (Alteneder & Hartzell 1997), following myocardial infarction (Seidl et al 1991) and spinal cord injury (Goddard 1988, Hodge 1995), as well as for clients undergoing haemodialysis (Gender 1999). The PLISSIT model is also promoted for use with individuals who have gynaecological conditions (Jolley 2002) as well as cancer (Smith 1989, Smith & Babaian 1992), multiple sclerosis (Nolan & Nolan 1998) and Hodgkin's disease (Cooley et al 1986).

The PLISSIT model is used widely and has been adopted by organisations such as the Royal College of Nursing (RCN) and the British Association of Sex and Relationship Therapists (BASRT). The literature shows extensive promotion of the PLISSIT model for use by nurses (Herson et al 1999, Royal College of Nursing 2000) and occupational therapists (Asrael 1985, McAlonan 1996). The model is by no means exclusive to these professions, for it has benefit for all health- and social-care professionals.

Asrael (1985, p. 3) asserts that 'every occupational therapist who is willing to regard the client as a human being has the skills and knowledge necessary to achieve the goals of the first two levels'. These skills are not unique to occupational therapists: 'anyone in the helping professions, regardless of job title, can provide some level of sexuality information' (Herson et al 1999, p. 149). Indeed, all practitioners who proclaim a holistic approach to care should address issues of sexuality and sexual health.

Before discussing the model in more depth and proposing an extension of the model, we will first clarify the terms 'sexuality' and 'sexual health'. The relevance of this model for all practitioners involved with rehabilitation will be considered in more detail as this chapter unfolds.

Sexuality and sexual health defined

It is a frequent misconception that sexuality is merely the expression of a physiological drive, resulting in sexual activity (Northcott & Chard 2000). While sexual behaviour is an element of sexuality, it is only one aspect. Sexuality is multifaceted (Hodge 1995), involving more than just the biological and physiological components of sexual behaviour and reproduction; it encompasses psychological and sociological aspects of how an individual relates to themselves and the world at large. The psychological aspects include a person's self-concept, self-esteem and body image, while sociological aspects include any religious and cultural factors and social roles (Meyer-Ruppel 1999).

Shope (1975, p. 3) suggests that sexuality involves, 'the total characteristics of an individual – social, personal and emotional – that are manifest in his or her relationships with others'. This is expressed in how we dress, how we feel about ourselves, our relationships and how we communicate with those around us (Medlar & Medlar 1990).

A similar definition is proposed by the Royal College of Nursing (2000, p. i), which defines sexuality as: 'an individual's self-concept, shaped by their personality and expressed as sexual feelings, attitudes, beliefs and behaviours, expressed through a heterosexual, homosexual, bisexual or transsexual orientation'. The need to identify differing sexual orientations within this definition is an explicit demonstration of inclusivity, the need for which results from the heterosexism that pervades our society.

Emphasising the all-pervading nature of sexuality, Stuart & Sundeen (1979) write, 'Sexuality is an integral part of the whole person. Human beings are sexual in every way, all the time. To a large extent human sexuality determines who we are. It is an integral factor in the uniqueness of every person.' This notion of sexuality is supported by Couldrick (1998, p. 493), who states that 'sexuality is an integral part of being human'.

Sexuality is a dynamic concept and is unique to each individual. An individual's sexuality changes in response to maturational, physiological, social and psychological events. Similarly, a medical diagnosis or admission to hospital will impinge on an individual's self-concept, self-esteem and social relationships. This in turn will affect their sexuality.

Recognising an individual's sexuality is an essential aspect of holistic care. The reason for taking sexuality into account in health care is to promote sexual health.

The World Health Organization (1975) defines sexual health as 'an integration of somatic, emotional, intellectual and social aspects of sexual being, in ways that are positive, enriching, and that enhance personality, communication and love'.

The Royal College of Nursing (2000, p. i) definition of sexual health is not dissimilar: 'the physical, emotional, psychological, social and cultural well being of a person's sexual identity, and the capacity and freedom to enjoy and express sexuality without exploitation, oppression, physical or emotional harm'.

Sexual health, therefore, is the freedom to express one's sexuality. Just as health is a matter of perception, where each person defines health differently, sexual health is also subjective. To one person, sexual health might mean freedom from infection; to another, sexual health is about feeling comfortable and secure within a relationship. To someone else, sexual health involves control of fertility; in terms either of preventing unplanned pregnancies or of becoming a parent. Each individual's notion of sexual health also changes over time. Sexuality and sexual health, therefore, are individual to each person and are deeply integrated in everyone's persona, clients and professionals alike.

The relevance of sexuality and sexual health for rehabilitation

Laflin (1996a) argues that the role of practitioners working in rehabilitation is to maximise each client's potential, despite any physical or emotional impairment. Indeed, 'if sexual behaviour is integral to a person's lifestyle, then part of rehabilitation is enabling the patient to adapt sexually' (Laflin 1996a, p. 367). Shell & Miller (1999, p. 53) are in agreement, stating that if the practitioner neglects to consider sexuality and sexual health as part of treatment and rehabilitation, this might result in the patient feeling 'less than human'. Other authors agree with this assertion, arguing that sexual health is a right (Wilson & McAndrew 2000) and that sexual adjustment is of major importance to individuals recovering from traumatic injury, disease or chronic illness (Miller 1984, Trombly 1989).

Many conditions can have an adverse effect on body image and self-worth, and have the potential to affect sexuality and sexual function. These include, but are not limited to, spinal cord injury, stroke, head injury, amputation, stomas, human immunodeficiency virus (HIV) infection, cancer, cardiac conditions, neurological conditions and even pregnancy.

The Royal College of Nursing (2000, p. 2) describes sexuality and sexual health as 'an appropriate and legitimate area of nursing activity' and does not restrict this assertion to any specific speciality. Similarly, Summerville & McKenna (1998, p. 275) state that 'sexuality education and counselling fall within the realms of legitimate occupational therapy'. Physiotherapists have a major role in the total rehabilitation process, and this is considered to incorporate sexual rehabilitation (Evans et al 1976, Summerville & McKenna 1998). Addressing issues relating to sexuality and sexual health are not exclusive to these three professional groups. While opinions vary in the literature as to the person *best* suited to address sexuality and sexual health needs, it is clear that the literature advocates a multidisciplinary approach (Evans et al 1976, Lemon 1993, Royal College of Nursing 2000).

Pearson et al (1996, p. 79), attempting to provide guidance on this important aspect of health, suggest that 'those aspects of sexuality relevant to the current need for nursing are explored'. The problem is, who decides what is relevant? The practitioner does not make decisions about what is relevant on behalf of the client in other aspects of rehabilitation. It is only through discussion and working in partnership with the client that goals are established and action plans formulated. The same should be true for issues relating to sexuality and sexual health.

Research studies show that clients do not voice their concerns about sexuality and sexual health because they feel vulnerable, shy and ashamed to ask (McAlonan 1996) and would prefer the professional to raise the subject first (Waterhouse 1996). In view of this, it becomes the responsibility of the practitioner to initiate discussion. Any lack of enquiry by the client should not be interpreted as a lack of concern about sexuality and sexual health (McAlonan 1996, Herson et al 1999, Shell & Miller 1999). The following sections provide guidance on how the practitioner can introduce the subject of sexuality and sexual health, and how the PLISSIT model can be used in practice.

Permission

There is some confusion in both the literature and clinical practice about the meaning of 'Permission' in the PLISSIT model. Some practitioners interpret this as *seeking* permission or consent from the client to discuss sexuality and sexual health issues. However, Annon (1976) was clear that Permission is an activity undertaken *by* the professional. To prevent confusion, it may be easier to use the term 'Permission-giving' to denote this first level of intervention.

Further confusion arises where authors define Permission as merely 'telling people that their thoughts, feelings and behaviours are normal' (Seidl et al 1991, p. 262) or 'giving [the client] permission to be sexual' (Herson et al 1999 p. 149). This is illustrated in the following extract: 'When Mrs Brown, who recently became paralysed, confides to her nurse that she still has sexual feelings, her nurse assures her that it is perfectly normal to continue to have sexual feelings, just like everyone else' (Herson et al 1999, p. 149).

In this example, the nurse has indicated to the client that there is nothing abnormal about her feelings. Through normalising sexuality, the nurse gives Permission for Mrs Brown to have sexual feelings. However, Mrs Brown is not necessarily given the opportunity to talk further about her sexuality. Permission-giving involves more than normalising sexuality, it also involves giving clients Permission to grieve for any loss (Summerville & McKenna 1998) and to discuss problems and concerns related to sexuality and sexual health (Royal College of Nursing 2000).

Practitioners need not be concerned that they have insufficient knowledge to function at this level. Irwin (2000, p.364) stresses that 'often patients will not expect the nurse to have the 'answer' to their problems . . . what a patient may require is the therapeutic space in which he or she can try to understand his or her feelings'. This involves creating an environment in which the client is able to voice any concerns or problems relating to their sexuality and sexual health. Privacy, dignity and safety are essential elements. Practitioners also need good listening skills and to be self-aware in order that they respect the values, beliefs and behaviour of clients.

When discussing sexual matters with clients, Bor & Watts (1993, p.659) provide clear guidance:

- Be purposeful
- Don't make assumptions
- Don't stereotype
- Ask questions
- Don't judge people
- Use the client's own words and language
- Remain professional
- Address relationships
- Ask when you don't understand a term or activity
- Address confidentiality, secrecy and privacy.

Pope (1997) recommends that sexual issues should be discussed in a 'matter of fact, non-judgmental way.' He argues that even a simple question such as 'Are you married?' indicates an assumption that all people are heterosexually orientated, since marriage *per se* is currently almost exclusively restricted by law to male–female couples. By adopting inclusive language, and recognising that sexuality and sexual health are relevant to everyone, practitioners should give Permission to clients to be sexual beings and to voice any questions, concerns or issues that they might have.

A frequent concern of health-care practitioners is the issue of timing. When is the right time to raise issues of sexuality and sexual health? Should it be done on admission, or is sexuality likely to be the last thing on the person's mind? Should it be discussed when planning for discharge, or left until after the individual has returned home?

A small-scale qualitative study by McAlonan (1996) explored the client's perspective on sexual rehabilitation services following spinal cord injury. Some individuals did think about the effects of their injury on relationships, sexual activity and fertility soon after their injury. However, all participants felt that they were not ready to address this aspect of rehabilitation immediately, 'but wanted to know that the information would be there when they were ready' (McAlonan 1996, p. 830).

One approach to Permission-giving involves asking cue questions so that individuals have the opportunity to raise any concerns they may have.

- 'People with cancer often have concerns or questions about how this will affect their sex life. Is there anything you'd like to ask me?'
- 'How has your incontinence affected the way you feel about yourself?' 'Has it affected the way you feel about yourself as a man/woman?'
- 'How is your relationship with your partner?' 'Has your condition affected your relationship in any way?' 'Would you like to talk about this?'

When asking questions such as these, the practitioner indicates to the client that sexuality is an important and appropriate topic for discussion. The practitioner also confirms that it is normal and appropriate to be sexual, to desire sexual activity and to discuss sexuality.

By giving the client Permission to discuss sexual issues, they are also given the opportunity to decline. It is important, therefore, that the practitioner is not intrusive and recognises any reluctance on the client's part. A word of caution is needed here, as there is a danger that the practitioner might interpret embarrassment and shyness as the client not wishing to talk about sexual matters. Any reluctance that is detected can be clarified with the question, 'Would you like to talk about this?'

If the client does not wish to discuss sexuality or sexual health, it is important to give them Permission to raise these issues at a later date.

- 'If you have any questions or concerns about sexuality later, do say and I'll do my best to help.'

In this way, the door is left open; clients are able to remain in control and make timely choices that best suit their needs.

ACTIVITY

- How might you ask about next of kin in an inclusive way?
- How might you ascertain whether an individual is sexually active?
- How might you ascertain the gender of an individual's sexual partner?

Friedman (1997) argues that Permission-giving should not be a one-off occurrence, as the importance of sexual issues to a client will vary in response to events such as after a home visit or before discharge. Therefore it is important that practitioners reiterate the Permission previously given in order to emphasise that the door remains open.

The aspects of Permission-giving that have been discussed so far all relate to the individual practitioner. However, White (2002, p. 249) extends this notion when she refers to creating a 'climate of Permission', which can occur at three key levels: the individual practitioner level, the level of systems of care delivery and the organisational level.

Establishing a climate of Permission at the organisational level

At the organisational level, White (2002) advocates sensitivity in recognising the need for private space, both for discussions between practitioners and clients and for clients to express their sexuality. Sherman (1999) cites an example that illustrates the importance of privacy in residential settings:

> *The Masons are in their 70s and, up to the time Mr Mason was admitted to the nursing home, they enjoyed a satisfactory sex life. Then he shared a room with three others and when Mrs Mason visited they walked together or sat beside his bed. Visitors were embarrassed when they came upon them in a passionate embrace. Moving Mr Mason into a single room gave them opportunities to be together undisturbed. Both were noticeably less stressed and his advances to female staff became rare.*
>
> *Sherman 1999, p. 99*

Further organisational factors discussed by White (2002) that influence Permission-giving include the organisational culture. This influences the availability of resources such as leaflets that promote sexual health, as well as reinforcing positive attitudes among staff.

A qualitative study conducted by Hitchcock & Wilson (1992) examined the factors influencing lesbian women to decide whether or not to disclose their sexual orientation to health-care providers, and their experiences as a consequence. Generating a theoretical understanding of the data, they suggest that individuals attempt to cope with the decision of whether or not to disclose their sexual orientation to a health-care professional through a process of 'personal risking'. This involves maintaining a psychologically safe environment as free as possible from reprisals and rejection.

The process of personal risking consists of two phases, the anticipatory and interactional phases. During the anticipatory phase, the risk of self-disclosure is considered using both imaginative and cognitive strategies. The individual considers the recommendations of friends and the particular health-care environment, and imagines the consequences of 'coming-out' to that health-care provider. In the interactional stage there is constant monitoring of the health-care provider's responses, again making use of both cognitive and emotional interpretation.

Understanding this process of personal risking is important for practitioners to identify ways to provide an environment in which it is safe for gay men, lesbian women and bisexuals to disclose their sexual identity. There is a need for visible evidence of a tolerant environment before individuals feel confident (Friedli 1989). Organisational strategies that give Permission in these circumstances include the provision of gay and lesbian literature and a space for sexual identity on forms, where so often the assumption is heterosexual.

This process of personal risking is not only of relevance to sexual identity. Before individuals disclose any sensitive information relating to sexuality or sexual health to practitioners, they are likely to weigh up the risks, based on both cognitive and emotional assessment. Individuals are more likely to feel safe and confident discussing sexual issues if the environment contains visible acknowledgement of individuals as sexual beings and acknowledges the need for privacy.

Establishing a climate of permission in systems of care delivery

It is important that systems of care delivery recognise and take into account factors that might impact on sexuality or sexual expression (White 2002). Permission-giving that takes place at the level of systems of care delivery includes recognising the need for flexibility and building this into packages of care. White (2002) gives the example of organising personal care at a time that suits the patient if there are particular times of day when sexual activity is easier or less tiring. Similarly, ensuring the provision of a care package that includes personal care if a man's partner finds that his feelings (e.g. when providing bowel care) intrude on their sexual relationship.

The development of assessment documentation that includes sexuality and sexual health as a core component is a useful system to facilitate Permission-giving. This inclusion enables practitioners to raise the topic of sexuality with clients as an integral aspect of their care (White 2002). It is, however, short-sighted to believe that, because sexuality is included in an assessment format, this aspect of care will be adequately addressed. Completed assessments that state 'likes to wear perfume' or 'married with one child' under this section are likely to indicate discomfort on the part of the practitioner and that this aspect of the assessment has not been adequately discussed with the client, if at all.

Continuity of staff is another element of care delivery at the systems level that may influence whether sexuality and sexual health issues are addressed. White (2002) recognises that care systems that promote continuity of staff, such as key worker or primary nursing systems, may strengthen relationships between practitioners and clients and may therefore be more conducive to clients disclosing or discussing sensitive issues. However, she also acknowledges that if a practitioner does not have the knowledge or skills to address these issues, or feels uncomfortable doing so, then the opportunities available to any clients in their care will be limited. White (2002) argues that staff must also be given Permission to discuss any discomfort or deficit in knowledge or skills with their line manager or in supervision.

Limited information

Providing information on sexuality and sexual health are important aspects of health care. 'Limited Information' refers to non-expert information (Royal College of Nursing 2000). However, in order to dispel myths and misconceptions about sexuality (McAlonan 1996), the practitioner does require sufficient knowledge about the impact of the condition, the medication prescribed and clinical intervention upon sexual wellbeing (White 2002). Limited Information may be given verbally, or in the form of a leaflet. It may also be given on an individual basis, to couples, or as part of a group process.

Both Hodge (1995) and Summerville & McKenna (1998) emphasise the element of Permission when giving Limited Information, advocating that the practitioner continue to convey Permission while providing information. It is therefore important not to restrict the open lines of communication that have begun at the Permission-giving level. This would happen if a leaflet were merely given to the client to read. A more helpful approach would be:

- 'There is a leaflet produced by the Stroke Association that talks about having sex after a stroke. Would you like to have a look at it? Then if you have any questions I would be happy to answer them.'

Using this approach, the practitioner can return to the topic at a later date:

- 'How helpful was the leaflet I gave you in answering questions about sexuality?'
- 'Was there anything that surprised you?'
- 'Do you have any further questions or concerns?'

A further example is a client who asks whether having an indwelling catheter will mean she can't have sex. The practitioner who responds appropriately would normalise the client's concern by stating that this is a frequent concern of people with catheters and provide information on how to manage the external devices at times of intimacy. Conveying information in this way responds to an individual's particular concern.

The Limited Information provided here differs from the next level of Specific Suggestion, as the Practitioner has not ascertained the client's current preferred sexual practices or identified her specific goals. Hence the general information that was provided was limited.

ACTIVITY

For your own area of practice, identify the following:
- What is the effect of the condition or treatment on sexuality and sexual health?
- How might you share this information with a client to normalise their experience?
- What client-information literature is available that addresses some of these issues?
- How might you respond to a question that you don't have the knowledge to answer?

Specific suggestions

To operate at the level of Specific Suggestions, the practitioner requires additional knowledge and skill (Royal College of Nursing 2000). The practitioner needs to take a sexual history and identify not only the problems but also the aspirations and expectations of the client (Seidl et al 1991). This level is based upon a problem-solving approach to address an individual's particular problem (Spica 1989).

Examples of Specific Suggestions include conception advice and the use of lubrication, sexual aids, contraception and alternative positions for sexual activity. The practitioner who has ascertained a client's concerns about sexual intercourse, for example, may provide advice on comfortable positions for sex for someone who has leg spasm as a consequence of multiple sclerosis, or is recovering from a stroke. This discussion may take place with or without the partner being present.

It is important to note that Specific Suggestions do not relate solely to sexual behaviour. As with all the levels of PLISSIT, all aspects of sexuality and sexual health are addressed. A client who says she is frightened that her partner will no longer find her attractive (since her surgery) may also be referring to her own sense of loss. The practitioner will need to assess how the woman herself perceives femininity and attractiveness, and how she displays this (perhaps through clothes, perfume, make-up, her hairstyle, etc.). Specific Suggestions will include discussion of those aspects that have meaning to this particular client and may result in referral for specialist intervention if the client is depressed as a result of this change in body image.

Intensive therapy

The most advanced level of PLISSIT requires specialist intervention as it involves complex interpersonal and psychological issues (Royal College of Nursing 2000). Laflin (1996b) and Herson et al (1999) recognise that specialist intervention is not only required to address relational or psychosexual issues but may also be required to address physical needs. Hence clients may require referral to a urologist or gynaecologist or may require relationship or psychosexual therapy.

Specific discussion of Intensive Therapy is beyond the scope of this chapter. It is important, however, that all practitioners are aware of sources of Intensive Therapy and are able to refer clients on. A selection of useful contact details is listed at the end of the chapter.

Limitations of PLISSIT

The linear format of the PLISSIT model implies a progression from one level to the next and does not recognise that a practitioner might need to return to previously addressed levels. This could result in practitioners feeling that they have addressed sexuality and sexual health once they have provided Limited Information. For example, when a practitioner informs a client who has joint or back pain that taking analgesia before any sexual activity would ensure optimum relief (Peate 2004) and might increase sexual participation (Laflin 1996b), the practitioner is implicitly indicating their own acceptance of sexual activity. This in itself is beneficial, as it gives the client Permission to be sexual and desire sexual activity. The client may be sufficiently reassured by this to feel able to voice their concerns. However, this is not a guarantee – the client may be uncertain whether it is appropriate to talk to this particular practitioner about their specific concerns. Unless practitioners give individuals Permission to *talk* about sexuality or sexual health and *discuss* their concerns, clients will remain uncertain. Implicit Permission-giving is inadequate, as individuals who feel embarrassed discussing sensitive issues will remain uncertain about the appropriateness of voicing their concerns. Permission-giving needs to be both explicit and unambiguous.

There is a further limitation of the PLISSIT model that is due to its linear format. Once practitioners have asked clients if they have any concerns or questions about how their condition will impact on their sexuality and sexual health, and given Permission to raise these concerns at any time, it would be easy to 'tick the box' and not return to sexual health issues again unless the client raises them. The danger here is that practitioners might feel that, since they have given Permission once, the client will be able to raise any further issues or concerns as they arise. This can result in the assumption that a lack of enquiry by the client indicates a lack of concern about sexuality and sexual health.

The PLISSIT model implies a one-way interaction in which the client is a passive recipient of a practitioner's interventions. While this was not Annon's (1976) intention, the practitioner may believe that they have given a client Permission and given Limited Information, yet without providing clients with an opportunity to engage in discussion and review the usefulness and appropriateness of the information given, this intervention is ineffective in meeting an individual's needs.

THE EX-PLISSIT MODEL

The Ex-PLISSIT model that is proposed here is an extension of the original PLISSIT model. White (2002) suggests that the four levels of intervention in the PLISSIT model are interconnected, although provides no further detail. The Ex-PLISSIT model develops this idea of interconnection further and consists of stages that can occur in any order (Fig. 6.1).

Given the attention we have paid so far to the level of Permission, it is perhaps unsurprising that each petal in the Ex-PLISSIT model has

Figure 6.1 The Ex-PLISSIT model promotes a comprehensive learning cycle of reflection and review, challenging assumptions in order to develop knowledge and self-awareness

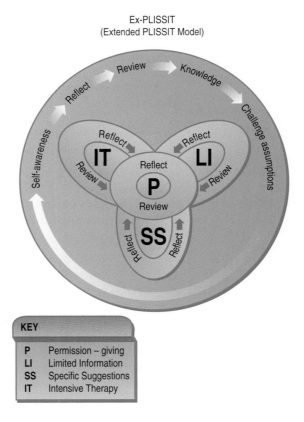

Ex-PLISSIT
(Extended PLISSIT Model)

KEY

P	Permission – giving
LI	Limited Information
SS	Specific Suggestions
IT	Intensive Therapy

ACTIVITY

Mr Khan is in a cardiac unit, recovering from a heart attack. His named nurse has been discussing discharge arrangements and giving advice about exercise.

The nurse gives him Permission to discuss issues relating to sexual health by saying, 'Do you have any questions or concerns about sexual activity when you go home?'

Mr Khan appears relieved and says 'Will it do any harm?'

The nurse provides a leaflet that provides information and reassurance about sexual activity following myocardial infarction and feels pleased that she has overcome her embarrassment and identified a problem that was quick and easy to address.

However:
- Is the client satisfied with the response?
- Has the leaflet answered all his questions?
- What are the range of issues and concerns that this client might potentially have?
- How might these be ascertained?

Permission-giving at its core. All interventions should begin with Permission, so each stage of Limited Information, Specific Suggestions and Intensive Therapy is underpinned by Permission-giving. It is important that practitioners maintain open lines of communication at all times so that clients feels able to raise any questions or concerns that they might have.

Unless the Permission-giving level is addressed first, the information that is given will be general and will not address the specific needs or concerns of the individual. For example, if the Limited Information given to a woman receiving radiotherapy focused on vaginal dryness, it would not meet the needs of a woman who regularly practised anal intercourse. The information that is given needs to be of relevance to the individual and the practitioner cannot assume that individuals will feel able to disclose *all* their issues and concerns at once. It is essential, therefore, that practitioners provide information that is inclusive and not restricted to assumptions made about the client's sexual preferences.

As stated previously, it is insufficient to provide a client with Limited Information without also providing an opportunity to review the usefulness and appropriateness of the information given. Meyer-Ruppel (1999) stresses that practitioners should not assume that once the topic has been discussed sexuality has been addressed and the issue is ended, for sexuality is a dynamic concept and issues will change in response to changes in physical, social and psychological circumstances. Integral within each stage of the Ex-PLISSIT model, therefore, are the principles of reflection and evaluation (review). These are made explicit at each stage.

In the example given, providing a client with a leaflet that contains information about sexual intercourse following a heart attack will not address concerns about a whole range of other issues such as masturbation, oral sex and current difficulties in maintaining an erection, to name but a few.

It is essential that practitioners reflect on their interactions and review the effectiveness of their interventions with clients. This process of review incorporates further Permission-giving as the client is given further opportunities to voice any issues that they might have. This can be done in the following way:

- 'How helpful was the leaflet I gave you in answering your questions about sexuality?'
- 'Was there anything that surprised you?'
- 'Do you have any further questions or concerns?'

This notion of on-going Permission-giving is not entirely new. Meyer-Ruppel (1999) encourages nurses working in gynae-oncology to consider questions about sexual health as routine, so that they are integral within the reassessment phase of each subsequent appointment. She does not refer to this questioning as Permission-giving as such, but it inevitably is.

Research indicates that practitioners believe that sexual rehabilitation is an essential aspect of rehabilitation; however, only a minority feel comfortable in discussing and addressing sexual issues (Ducharme & Gill 1990, Katz & Aloni 1999, Haboubi & Lincoln 2003). This conflict between practitioners' ideology and practice is indicative of the discomfort that many feel in discussing sexuality and sexual health.

ACTIVITY

Identify other ways in which you can give clients Permission to raise the topic of sexuality and sexual health at a later date.

Herson et al (1999, p. 149) argue that the most important quality a practitioner needs in addressing sexual health issues is 'personal comfort regarding sexuality and disability'. Hodge (1995) suggests that Permission also involves giving the *practitioner* Permission to refer the client on to another professional. This recognition that individual practitioners are not required to function at all levels is a strength of PLISSIT, ensuring that practitioners operate within their own level of comfort. However, unless reflection and review are undertaken, which enhance knowledge, challenge assumptions and increase self-awareness, practitioners will not progress or develop. These elements of reflection and review are integral to the Ex-PLISSIT model, ensuring ongoing learning and development.

Reflection and self-awareness are key components of effective interactions with clients. To achieve a level of personal comfort, Laflin (1996b) encourages practitioners to examine their own attitudes and beliefs in order to be able to provide sexual information in a non-judgemental way.

Research undertaken with individuals who have a spinal cord injury identified qualities of health-care practitioners that influenced their own receptiveness, confidence, the amount of disclosure and level of satisfaction with sexuality information received during rehabilitation (McAlonan 1996). One participant described his experience with a nurse practitioner: '[She] was very good . . . easy to talk to . . . [with her], it's no big deal, it's part of life, same as bowel care, bladder care, something you have to deal with '(McAlonan 1996, p. 829).

Approachability, empathy, willingness to listen and an adequate comfort level are the qualities described by McAlonan (1996) as essential.

In the PLISSIT model, Summerville & McKenna (1998, p. 278) indicate that Intensive Therapy is provided 'when intervention via the lower three levels has not been effective'. The Ex-PLISSIT model indicates that Intensive Therapy may be offered at *any* stage. For example, a client may be given Permission to discuss sexuality through the provision of Limited Information:

- 'Are you aware that impotence is a side effect of these tablets?'

The client may respond by stating that he has been impotent for some time, even before he began taking these tablets. If he wishes to address this problem, it would be appropriate to refer him for further assessment without first passing through the stage of Specific Suggestions.

Similarly, if having given the client Permission, the practitioner is challenged with something they feel completely unable to deal with, then it should be possible for them to suggest referral to Intensive Therapy without passing through the other stages first.

Applications for use

While the PLISSIT model was originally developed to address issues in relation to sexuality and sexual health, there is no reason why it cannot be used for other aspects of health and social care provision. Similarly, we would advocate using the Ex-PLISSIT model when addressing other sensitive areas such as issues of loss and adaptation in rehabilitation.

REHABILITATION

This section will consider in more detail the implications of the Ex-PLISSIT model for rehabilitation practitioners. As already discussed, the PLISSIT model has been used extensively in the literature and in practice to address the sexuality and sexual health needs of clients. Although there is possibly a use for it in dealing with other sensitive areas, there is a real issue with clients' sexuality and sexual health-care needs not being addressed adequately in rehabilitation. This section will therefore discuss the use of the Ex-PLISSIT model in addressing a client's sexuality and sexual health needs in rehabilitation.

When thinking about terminology it is useful to consider whether there is a more encompassing term that can be used when considering a client's sexuality and sexual health needs in rehabilitation. In 2004, a working party at the regional brain injury unit at Northwick Park Hospital considered clients' sexuality and sexual health-care needs and agreed on the term 'sexual wellbeing' as being conducive to the concept of rehabilitation. Wellbeing can be identified as encompassing all those domains that make up a 'good life'. These include physical, mental and social aspects (World Health Organization 2001). Wellbeing can also be about how one is feeling and can be equated to a high level of self-esteem.

When considering health promotion and rehabilitation, Davis (1999) identifies that clients going through the rehabilitation process generally have low self-esteem because of their loss of control of their lives and that ultimately rehabilitation should therefore be aiming to increase their level of control and ultimately their level of wellbeing. Being more specific in using the term 'sexual wellbeing' may help to ensure that sexuality and sexual health care are addressed explicitly, at the same time putting it in the context of wellbeing generally for each individual. Sexual wellbeing fits in well with the notion of rehabilitation being concerned with the totality of the person with the ultimate aim of maximising an individual's quality of life. For this section of the chapter the term sexual wellbeing will be used to encompass sexuality and sexual health-care needs for clients going through the rehabilitation process.

ICF or International Classification of Functioning, Disability and Health

The link between the Ex-PLISSIT model and the ICF is that Ex-PLISSIT as an intervention model is an ideal framework to address some of the more sensitive areas that are identified in the ICF (World Health Organization 2001). Sexual wellbeing, which has been the focus of the PLISSIT model in the literature, is acknowledged in the ICF in terms of contextual factors as well as functioning and disability. The ICF identifies different categories that relate to sexual wellbeing (Box 6.1).

One of the strengths of the ICF is its comprehensive inclusion of a number of areas that contribute to an individual's wellbeing. In including the above categories it has acknowledged the integral part sexuality and sexual health play for an individual. It considers issues of sexual wellbeing in terms of:

Box 6.1   ICF Categories Related to Sexual Wellbeing

Body Functions

Chapter 1: Mental function; Chapter 6: Genitourinary and reproductive functions.
b1801: 'Body Image: Specific mental functions related to the representation and awareness of one's own body' (p. 61)
b6400: 'Functions of sexual arousal phase: functions of sexual interest and excitement' (p. 90)
b6401: 'Functions of sexual preparatory phase: functions of engaging in sexual intercourse' (p. 90)
b6402: 'Functions of orgasmic phase: functions of reaching orgasm' (p. 90)
b6403; 'Functions of sexual resolution phase: functions of satisfaction after orgasm and accompanying relaxation' (p. 91)

Activities and Participation

Chapter 7: Interpersonal interactions and relationships
d7100: 'Respect and warmth in relationships: showing and responding to consideration and esteem, in a contextually and socially appropriate manner' (p. 159)
d7105: 'Physical contact in relationships: making and responding to bodily contact with others, in a contextually and socially appropriate manner' (p. 159)
d7702: 'Sexual relationships: creating and maintaining a relationship of a sexual nature, with a spouse or other partner' (p. 163)

Environmental Factors

Chapter 4: Attitudes
e450: 'Individual attitudes of health professionals: general or specific opinions and beliefs of health care professionals about the person or about other matters (e.g. social, political and economic issues) that influence individual behaviour and actions' (p. 191)
e465: 'Social norms, practice and ideologies: customs, practices, rules and abstract systems of values and normative beliefs (e.g. ideologies, normative world views and moral philosophies) that arise within social contexts and that affect or create societal and individual practices and behaviours, such as social norms of moral and religious behaviour or etiquette; religious doctrine and resulting norms and practices; norms governing rituals or social gatherings' (p. 191)

- *Body image*: the way individuals feel about their body and the awareness they have of their own body. The ICF doesn't categorise self-image or self-concept
- *Physical functions related to the sexual act*: The phases of the act are highlighted, from arousal to resolution. Categorising physical functions in this way can perhaps help clients and rehabilitation professionals feel more comfortable in acknowledging that the sexual act is a legitimate function
- *Interpersonal interactions and relationships*: The ICF categorises a number of different personal interactions in different contexts that include formal relationships, informal social relationships, family relationships and intimate relationships. This highlights the importance of relationships in a variety of contexts for an individual's wellbeing
- *Attitudes*: As already mentioned earlier on in this chapter, attitudes, values and beliefs all play an important part in the way clients' sexual wellbeing needs are met by health-care professionals. The ICF categorises attitudes in terms of individuals, friends, acquaintances, health-care professionals, personal care providers and personal assistants. It also identifies the importance of social norms and practices.

The ICF in its identification of categories that relate to an individual's sexual wellbeing could be used to structure rehabilitation professionals' interventions at the different stages in the Ex-PLISSIT model. The ICF categories could be used as cues for rehabilitation professionals to ensure that they are considering an individual's sexual wellbeing. For example, the different categories around relationships could be used as a guide to ensure that these are considered. These may need to be considered at all stages.

The ICF categories could be used to develop an assessment tool that could be used at each stage. Using the ICF and the Ex-PLISSIT model to complement each other could enable the rehabilitation team to identify categories they need to consider in relation to a client's sexual wellbeing. Team members could then identify the stage of the Ex-PLISSIT model they feel comfortable with rather than thinking that they need individually to address all categories. Using both models together could help promote a team approach rather than the team considering clients' sexual wellbeing to be the province of one professional group.

The Ex-PLISSIT model identifies that, although the process needs to start at the Permission-giving stage, Intensive Therapy can be offered at any stage. The model embeds the whole process within a learning cycle of reflection and review that highlights the need for the team to reflect and review as a team as well as individually.

The role of the team

Interprofessional working is fundamental in rehabilitation whether the team approach is multi-disciplinary or inter-disciplinary. The focus needs to be on goals the clients have themselves identified as being important to them. As already highlighted it is important that addressing clients' sexual wellbeing is seen as the role of the whole team. The Ex-PLISSIT model with its focus on levels of intervention can be used to help the team identify how they can best work together. In this section a case study identified initially in chapter two will be used to illustrate how this might work in practice.

CASE STUDY JOEY

Joey is a 50 year old single unemployed man who lives with his partner, John. Joey is in hospital recovering from a heart attack. Before the heart attack Joey led generally a sedentary lifestyle, going out only to go to the shops. His relationship with John was strong and they had an active sexual relationship. The team are now preparing for Joey to be discharged. Joey is very anxious about this and worried about his relationship with John. He feels that John doesn't find him attractive any more.

The team have been discussing Joey's discharge plans and have identified his anxiety about going home. One of the nurses has noticed that Joey is quite abrupt with John and won't let him touch him. The team discuss whether there may be some issues for Joey in terms of his relationship with John. Some of the team express their anxieties at having to discuss this with John and question whether it is their role. There is some general discussion, facilitated by Mary, the clinical specialist nurse, who does address sexual wellbeing with clients. This leads to the team reflecting on their role and results in them agreeing that Joey needs to feel that he can discuss his anxieties in terms of his relationship with John. He needs 'Permission' to do this. There is some discussion about whether this should include John, but it is felt that Joey needs to have the opportunity to discuss his concerns first. Involving John at this stage without Joey's consent could cause irreparable damage. Some members feel that Mary should address this with Joey, but Mary feels that, although she knows Joey, she has had limited contact with him. Sheila, the occupational therapist, has already organised a meeting with Joey to discuss his home situation in light of his discharge. She feels comfortable about raising the issue of sexuality with Joey.

In this meeting, which is held in a private office, Sheila asks Joey if he has any concerns over his relationship with John when he goes home. Joey then begins to talk about his feelings of unattractiveness and the fact that John won't physically touch him. Sheila is able to use cue questions and prompts to encourage Joey to discuss his feelings. As the meeting progresses she is also able to ask Joey specifically about sexual activity with John. At this point Joey feels comfortable with expressing his worries about this side of his and John's relationship. Sheila is able to reassure Joey that what he is feeling is a normal reaction to his heart attack.

However, Sheila recognises that Joey would benefit from more explicit Information and Specific Suggestions about sexual activity after a heart attack. She feels that she doesn't have the knowledge to deal with this aspect, so she asks Joey if he would feel comfortable talking about these issues with Mary, who has more experience in this area. Sheila offers to sit in with Joey if he wants. Joey agrees to this.

In order to increase Joey's self-esteem, Sheila also negotiates with him some activities in his occupational therapy sessions that involve him socialising with other people. Sheila suggests to Joey that he might like to have clothes brought in from home, which he could wear on the ward, and that she could arrange for him to have his hair cut if he wants that. Sheila also suggests that Joey might like to have some quiet time with John before discharge by going out from the ward with John.

At the meeting with Mary and Sheila, Mary is able to give Joey some Specific Suggestions about resuming sexual activity after the heart attack. She also gives Joey a leaflet that reinforces what she has said. Mary suggests that Joey might like to show the leaflet to John and that she will be happy to talk to both of them. Joey agrees to this and asks if Sheila will tell John about their meeting and the subsequent meeting with Mary. Sheila agrees to do this with Joey present. Sheila fells that it will be useful to feed back generally to the team and she gets consent from Joey to do this.

At the next team meeting the team reflects on whether they could have given Joey Permission earlier to discuss his concerns. Sheila's experience with Joey enables her and the team to reflect on how they address clients' sexual wellbeing. They realise that, although they do have leaflets on display they don't prompt clients to read them or follow them up with discussion. The team also identifies that in the past they have perhaps tended to rely on Mary to address clients' sexual wellbeing, whereas she may not always be the appropriate person for the initial meeting.

It is useful to consider the case study of Joey in terms of the stages of the Ex-PLISSIT model and how they occurred.

Stage 1: Permission-giving

In the above example, the different stages can clearly be seen. If the nurse had not picked up on Joey's anxiety and discussed it at a team meeting then Joey could have been discharged without discussing his anxieties. The fact that the team had regular team meetings and obviously felt comfortable with each other enabled members of the team to express their anxieties without feeling they were being judged. This is also Permission-giving for the team and is vital if the team are to reflect, evaluate and develop self-awareness. Sheila identified the stage she felt comfortable with and perhaps the reason she felt comfortable to address the issues with Joey was because she saw it as a natural element of discharge planning. The way Sheila brought in the topic gave Joey Permission to discuss it. Joey was also able to see that it was important to discuss in terms of going home. Because Sheila discussed the subject in relation to going home it was discussed in context.

Stage 2: Limited Information

Limited Information was given to Joey verbally when Sheila explained what could be expected following a heart attack. Sheila was going to give Joey a leaflet to read but, because of Joey's anxieties, she felt that it might increase them. On reflection, Sheila decided that it would be more useful for Joey to talk to Mary and for Mary to give him written information. As Joey was discussing his sexual wellbeing with Sheila, she was constantly giving him Permission to discuss more intimate issues, i.e. his sexual activity.

Stage 3: Specific Suggestions

Sheila made Specific Suggestions regarding Joey's feelings of unattractiveness. Sheila recognised that Joey's main anxiety was about John not wanting him any more and not finding him attractive. By suggesting opportunities for increased social interactions and suggesting ways for Joey to feel more comfortable with his image, e.g. wearing his own clothes, having his hair cut, Sheila anticipated that these might help to increase Joey's confidence in himself.

During the meeting with Mary, Mary took a sexual history from Joey that was based on the categories in the ICF. This meant that she covered sexual functions, relationships and attitudes. This enabled her to identify Joey's current sexual practices, his aspirations and expectations. By doing this she was able to identify what the problems were for Joey. As a result of this Mary gave Joey Specific Suggestions based on the current literature on sexual activity after a heart attack. For example, anal intercourse can have an impact on coronary health in the recovery period due to stimulation of the vagus nerve, which may cause chest pain (McCann 1989, cited in Crumlish 2004). Mary suggested to Joey that, even though it would be safer not to have anal sexual intercourse while he was recovering, he could still participate in other sexual activities. Mary was also able to reduce Joey's anxieties about positions for sexual activity, as he had heard that it was better after a heart attack to sit on a chair for sexual intercourse. Mary was able to reassure him that evidence had now shown that this is not the case (Crumlish 2004). Any position was fine as long as it was comfortable for him and John.

Stage 2: Limited Information

Mary gave Joey a leaflet, which could be seen as giving Limited Information, but she used it to reinforce her Specific Suggestions. Mary also used the leaflet as a way for Joey to involve John in the discussion.

Stage 1: Permission-giving

Again during stage 3, when Mary gave information and Specific Suggestions she was giving Joey Permission to ask quite intimate questions. The leaflet can also be seen as a way for Joey to give John Permission to discuss his concerns.

Stage 3: Specific Suggestions

In the subsequent meeting with Joey and John, Mary repeated the specific advice and Specific Suggestions she had already talked to Joey about.

Stage 4: Intensive Therapy

One of the actions that might come out of the meeting with Joey, John and Mary is for Mary to make Joey and John aware that there is more intensive counselling available if they would like it. Joey might find counselling useful in terms of his relationship with John or in terms of his own feelings about feeling unattractive. This referral may not be made until Joey has been home for a while, as the issue may not become evident until then. Mary or Sheila could continue to act as a link after Joey goes home.

Learning cycle

In terms of the learning cycle, which is a vital element of the Ex-PLISSIT model, it is apparent that Sheila reflected on the information she was getting from Joey and that it was this reflection that directed her actions. The team were able to challenge and discuss their own assumptions at that first team meeting and also to reflect on and evaluate their subsequent interactions with Joey. As a result, they identified some actions that they could take in terms of creating Permission for clients. If sexual wellbeing for clients is to be an integral element of rehabilitation then it is vital that this learning cycle takes place.

The example of Joey illustrates the importance of the whole team being involved in meeting a client's sexual wellbeing. Mary used the ICF to assess Joey's sexual wellbeing; however, the team could also use the categories to enable them to consider clients' sexual wellbeing more consistently. The above example also highlights how the level of Permission is an integral element of each stage.

Issues to consider

There are a number of specific issues that arise from the case study that need to be considered when using the Ex-PLISSIT model in relation to rehabilitation. These are also supported by research studies considering the sexual wellbeing of different client groups. Table 6.1 gives a brief overview of some of these studies. Although these studies are all limited in terms of their generalisability – for example, they use small numbers of participants – they do come up with similar findings and implications for using the Ex-PLISSIT model.

Privacy

Mayers & Heller (2003) make the point that the degree of privacy may dictate the level clients can progress to. Sheila and Mary considered carefully where their meetings should take place and they planned them so that they wouldn't be disturbed. Privacy is an issue for all stages of the Ex-PLISSIT model.

Gender

One issue to consider at all stages is the importance the client places on their gender role. Guttman and Napier-Klemic (1995) found that men may feel inadequate if they are unable to resume their role as a man. This wasn't an issue raised explicitly by Joey but it is perhaps important for rehabilitation professionals to consider that this may be an issue. It may

Table 6.1 Research studies and their link to the Ex–PLISSIT model

Sample and Aim	Findings	Links to Ex–PLISSIT
Guttman & Napier-Klemic 1995 The experience of head injury on the impairment of gender identity and gender role		
Two males and two females. *Aim*: to examine the disruption of gender identity and gender role as a result of traumatic brain injury	The men relied more heavily on traditional gender-specific activities before and after injury to define themselves as a man; they expressed feelings of inadequacy if they were unable to resume these activities	Highlights the importance of considering how individuals see themselves in terms of their gender. This may have implications for who individuals will feel comfortable with in terms of discussing their sexual wellbeing
Mayers & Heller 2003 Sexuality and the late-stage Huntington's disease patient		
Four males and five females in a residential care home. *Aim*: to identify any sexual issues and individuals' perceptions of their ultimate and sexual relationships	Caregivers need to recognise that patients are sexual beings with sexual needs, fantasies and wishes by providing: privacy; sexually orientated videos or reading materials; romance novels or films; the means for individuals to stimulate themselves	Supports the need for privacy which is a prerequisite for all levels. The degree of privacy in a care home situation may dictate the level patients can progress to. Supports the use of providing sexually related material and sexual aids which relates to stage 3
Westgren & Levi 1999 Sexuality after injury: interviews with women after traumatic spinal cord injury		
Eight women. *Aim*: to illuminate the women's sexual experiences. *Explored*: first sexual contact after injury; communication with partner before and after injury; sexual activity after injury	Strong influence of pre-injury sexual behaviour on post-injury adaptation. A positive outlook and good communication skills were linked to a favourable rehabilitation outcome	Supported the need for psychological support and practical advice after discharge. This highlights the need for stage 3, where practical advice would be given, and stage 4, where more specialist support is required
Mona et al 2000 Sexual expression following spinal cord injury		
109 men and 86 women. *Aim*: to explore sexual adjustment through cognitive adaptation theory	Rehabilitation professionals can provide better treatment planning and interventions if they have a deeper understanding of the psychological variables associated with positive adjustment	Treatment suggestions included giving patients permission to talk about sexuality; normalising the experience for patients; giving information; referring patients on. These all relate to all stages in Ex-PLISSIT
Edmans 1998 An investigation of stroke patients resuming sexual activity		
Six males, six females, nine partners. *Aim*: to identify whether they had been able to resume their sexual activity and what information they would find useful	Lack of interest/motivation, physical difficulties and difficulties in arousal identified as the main problems faced by the participants in relation to rehabilitation	Highlights the importance of the stages of Permission-giving and Limited Information. The participants wanted information when they started to spend time at home at weekends and before discharge

Sample and Aim	Findings	Links to Ex-PLISSIT
Taleporos & McCabe 2002 The impact of sexual esteem, body esteem, and sexual satisfaction on psychological well-being in people with physical disability		
A comparison of 748 participants with a physical disability and 448 without. *Aim*: to compare sexual well-being with psychological well being	Sexual esteem, body esteem, and sexual satisfaction are strong predictors of self-esteem and depression for people with a physical disability. Body esteem more associated with women and sexual esteem with men	Identifies the need for the identification of strategies to improve the body esteem and sexual wellbeing of people with physical disabilities

also be an issue for women, in terms of not being able to resume their role as a partner/mother.

Normalising the experience

Mona et al (2000) talk about normalising the experience for patients. Sheila did this with Joey by reassuring him that what he was feeling was a normal reaction following a heart attack. It is important for clients to see that problems they may have regarding their sexual wellbeing are not abnormal and that other clients have similar issues. This needs to happen in stage 1, as it is a way of creating Permission for clients to discuss their sexual wellbeing.

Providing sexual aids

Mayers & Heller (2003) talk about using sexually-related videos and reading material as well as sexual aids. Giving practical suggestions is also supported by Westgren & Levi (1999). This reinforces stage 3, giving Specific Suggestions, a stage that not all rehabilitation professionals may feel comfortable with. Sheila identified that she didn't feel comfortable at stage 3 because of her lack of knowledge, which is why she involved Mary. In rehabilitation, the provision of aids of daily living is a key feature for some clients; perhaps this should include the provision of sexual aids, if that is identified as a need for a client's sexual wellbeing.

Context

In Edmans' (1998) study, participants wanted information when they started to spend time at home. Joey felt comfortable discussing issues with Sheila because he could see how it related to him being discharged. This highlights the importance of discussing clients' sexual wellbeing in context and that is why it is vital that it is a team endeavour. Examples of this are:

- Nurses discussing sexual activity when discussing continence with a client
- Physiotherapists discussing positions for sex when discussing sleeping positions
- Occupational therapists discussing body image when talking about washing and dressing

- Doctors and nurses discussing the effects of medication on a client's sexual wellbeing – although this can be seen as a stage 2 intervention, as it is giving information, it may also open the way for more in-depth discussion that not all professionals would feel comfortable with
- The team discussing sleeping arrangements when conducting a home visit and exploring the effects of this on a client's relationship. This may result in suggestions of exploring alternative methods of achieving sexual satisfaction.

It can make it more difficult for the rehabilitation professional and the client if it feels like a special time has been arranged to discuss sexual issues, although this may be appropriate if it is an agreed arrangement from a previous meeting. Discussing sexual wellbeing in context will have an effect on the level of comfortableness for the client and the rehabilitation professional and can be seen as contributing to stage 1: Permission-giving.

Developing strategies

Taleporos & McCabe (2002) identify the importance of health-care professionals developing strategies to improve clients' body image and self-esteem. This was a major issue for Joey in that he felt unattractive and insecure. Sheila was able to identify strategies that would help him.

The studies in Table 6.1 and the case study of Joey reinforce the stages of Ex-PLISSIT and the need for reflection and review. They also highlight the importance of using an interprofessional approach to address clients' sexual wellbeing. None of the studies indicated that this was the role of a specific professional group.

Examples from practice

The following two accounts are examples of how the PLISSIT model is being used in rehabilitation settings.

Example 1: Sexual wellbeing policy and guidelines

This policy was developed in 2004 by J. Johnson, J. Thrilling, J. Gregory and F. Gawn in the Regional Rehabilitation Unit at Northwick Park Hospital in response to the rehabilitation professionals wanting to improve practice with regards to clients' sexual wellbeing. A working party was formed, and agreed on the term 'sexual wellbeing' for reasons discussed earlier in this chapter. The unit's policy covers:

- The unit's philosophy that sexual wellbeing is an important aspect of rehabilitation. It includes subscribing to the PLISSIT model to guide the level of staff involvement and, as a result, provide a framework for staff education at various stages
- Confidentiality, including disclosure of information and breaching confidentiality
- Abuse: within the unit's philosophy, sexual abuse is defined as involvement in sexual activities which an individual does not want or has not consented to or cannot understand or is unable to consent to
- Approaches to sexual wellbeing in the unit. The policy identifies two main approaches depending on whether sexual behaviour needs to

be rehabilitated or is an unwelcome/inappropriate consequence of brain injury. The PLISSIT model is used to guide these approaches
● Various resources, including a list of Regional Rehabilitation Unit staff able to work at PLISSIT stages 2 and 3, as well as more specialist referrals at stage 4 within and outside the Trust.

The policy identifies flow charts to guide responses at stages 1 and 2 (Figs 6.2, 6.3). These flow charts give inexperienced members of the team guidance on how to operate at stages 1 and 2. They help ensure some consistency among the team and, as well as giving all patients Permission to raise sexual wellbeing issues in rehabilitation, they give staff Permission to identify the stage they feel happy and confident with.

Using the Ex-PLISSIT model would add in the element of reflection and self-awareness for staff. Although the flow charts implicitly incorporate reflection and review at each stage as the rehabilitation professional has to go through these processes in order to make a decision about the next stage.

Example 2: Relationship and Sexual Issues Questionnaire

A working party was formed in 2004 at the Oxford Centre for Enablement, Oxford, in response to nurses' anxieties about addressing issues of sexuality and sexual health with clients. As a result of the working party two questionnaires were developed by S Hunt and J Parra to give the team

Figure 6.2 Sexually related enquiries: guidance for a response at level 1 of PLISSIT (from Northwick Park Regional Rehabilitation Unit Philosophy, 2004)

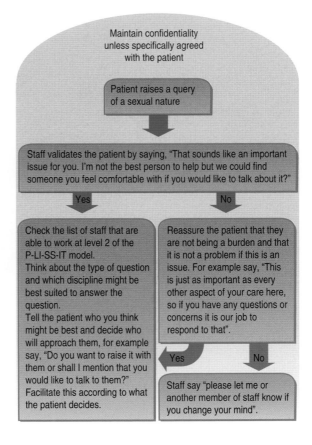

Figure 6.3 Sexually related enquiries: guidance for a response at level 2 of PLISSIT (from Northwick Park Regional Rehabilitation Unit Philosophy, 2004)

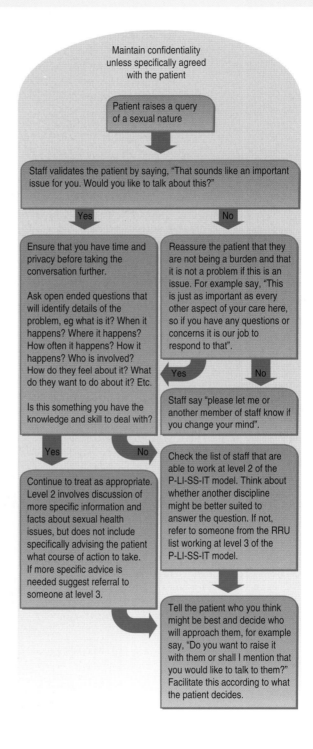

Permission to address clients' sexual wellbeing: one for clients with partners and one for clients without partners (Boxes 6.2, 6.3). The questionnaire is usually completed 2–3 weeks after the client's admission, when they are asked to consider their life goals. In the unit, life goals are used to enable client-centred goal planning. The questionnaire is usually facilitated by a trained nurse or a health-care assistant, depending on the relationship between the client and the nurse. One of the issues for the unit is that dealing with clients' sexual wellbeing is generally seen by the team as the nurse's role. The team includes a psychosexual doctor whom clients can be referred to. The team have also developed a booklet about *Sexual Health and Relationships*, which is used to give clients Permission to discuss issues.

Both these examples from practice show how developing different strategies and tools can help with the implementation of the Ex-PLISSIT model.

Using the Ex-PLISSIT model to develop a training programme

It is important that all of the team feel prepared to operate at stages 1 and 2. The team then need to identify those professionals who feel comfortable with stage 3. This highlights the need for training at each stage. The Ex-PLISSIT model can be used to structure a training programme to the rehabilitation team at each stage:

- *Stage 1: Permission-giving*
  - Re-visiting communication skills: paraphrasing; listening; picking up on cues; transactional analysis
  - Looking at the use of language
  - Identifying some core cue questions that can be used with the team's client group

---

Box 6.2   Relationship and Sexual Issues Questionnaire: patients without a partner

1. Have you ever had a partner?
2. Was it a sexual relationship?
3. Do you have any thoughts or concerns about future relationships or sexual needs?
4. Would you like some more information or would you like to meet with someone, in confidence, to discuss any of the above issues?

Source: Oxford Centre for Enablement (2004)

Box 6.3   Relationship and Sexual Issues Questionnaire: patients with a partner

1. Do you have a partner?
2. How long have you been together?
3. Has your relationship changed since your illness/stroke?
4. How has it changed?
5. What was it like before?
6. Has your sexual relationship changed?
7. How has it changed?
8. Would you like some more information or would you like to meet with someone, in confidence, to discuss any of the above issues?

Source: Oxford Centre for Enablement (2004)

- Using exercises to enable the team to consider their own attitudes, values and beliefs.
- *Stage 2: Limited Information*
  - How to use written information
  - Looking at the type of written information available for the specific client group
  - Identifying the types of Limited Information that may be appropriate to give at this level for the particular client group
- *Stage 3: Specific Suggestions.* At this level more specific knowledge will be needed regarding the following areas:
  - Sexual assessment
  - Normal sexual function
  - Sexual dysfunction
  - Sexual positions
  - Incontinence and sexual activity
  - The use of sexual aids.
- *Stage 4: Intensive Therapy.* Although clients are referred on at this level it is still important that rehabilitation professionals know what this level entails so that they can refer on knowledgeably. It might be useful for specialists to talk to the team about their role.

At each stage enabling staff to reflect on practice and on their own feelings is important. It may be useful to re-introduce a reflective framework (Johns & Freshwater 1998), which can be used to promote the learning cycle that is key to the Ex-PLISSIT model. The learning cycle can also be used by the team consistently to reflect on and review the sexual wellbeing of specific clients and issues that may arise.

CONCLUSION

This chapter has critically discussed the use of the PLISSIT model and its limitations. In light of this, an extended model Ex-PLISSIT, was outlined and discussed in relation to rehabilitation. This chapter has focused on the use of PLISSIT and Ex-PLISSIT in addressing clients' sexual wellbeing, although it could also be used to address other sensitive issues.

There are obvious links between the Ex-PLISSIT model and the ICF, and indeed using these two frameworks together can help rehabilitation professionals identify how as a team they can address clients' sexual wellbeing. The case study of Joey identified how Ex-PLISSIT could be used in practice by the whole team and highlighted the fact that the stages of Ex-PLISSIT are not necessarily followed in order and that Permission-giving is integral to each stage. The examples from practice gave an idea of the kinds of strategy that can be developed to assist in implementing Ex-PLISSIT. Training is essential if rehabilitation professionals are to use it effectively in practice and the suggested training programme shows how Ex-PLISSIT can also help to determine the content of such a programme.

QUESTIONS FOR PRACTICE

- How as a team do you address clients' sexual wellbeing?
- How could you use the Ex-PLISSIT model as a team?
- Using the Ex-PLISSIT model, identify the training needs you need as a team to address each stage
- How might you use the ICF and Ex-PLISSIT together?

References

Annon J 1976 The PLISSIT model: a proposed conceptual scheme for the behavioural treatment of sexual problems. Journal of Sex Education Therapy 2:1–15

Asrael W 1985 The PLISSIT model of sexuality counselling and education. Physical Disabilities Special Interest Section Newsletter 8(2):3–4

Alteneder R, Hartzell D 1997 Addressing couples' sexuality concerns during the childbearing period: use of the PLISSIT model. Journal of Obstetric, Gynecologic and Neonatal Nursing 26:651–658

Bor R, Watts M 1993 Talking to clients about sexual matters. British Journal of Nursing 2:657–661

Cooley M, Yeomans A, Cobb S 1986 Sexual and reproductive issues for women with Hodgkin's disease II. Application of PLISSIT Model. Cancer Nursing 9:248–255

Couldrick L 1998 Sexual issues: an area of concern for occupational therapists. British Journal of Occupational Therapy 61:493–496

Crumlish B 2004 Sexual counselling by cardiac nurses for patients following an MI. British Journal of Nursing 13:710–713

Davis S M 1999 The relationship between health promotion and rehabilitation. In: Davis S, O'Connor S (eds) Rehabilitation nursing: foundations for practice. Baillière Tindall, London

Davis S M 2004 The relationship between health promotion and rehabilitation. In: Davis S, O'Connor S 2004 (eds) Rehabilitation nursing: foundations for practice, 4th edn. Baillière Tindall, Edinburgh

Ducharme S, Gill K 1990 Sexual values, training and professional roles. Journal of Head Trauma Rehabilitation 5:38–45.

Edmans J 1998 An investigation of stroke patients resuming sexual activity. British Journal of Occupational Therapy 61:36–38

Evans R, Haler E, deFreece A et al 1976 Multidisciplinary approach to sex education of spinal cord injured patients. Physical Therapy 56:541–545

Friedli L 1989 Promoting our health. Conference Report. Oxford City Council, Oxford

Friedman J 1997 Sexual expressions: the forgotten component of ADL. OT Practice 2:20–25

Gender A 1999 Clinical implications of sexual dysfunction in men on chronic haemodialysis. Rehabilitation Nursing 24:27

Goddard L 1988 Sexuality and spinal cord injury. Journal of Neuroscience Nursing 20:240–244

Guttman SA, Napier-Klemic J 1995 The experience of head injury on the impairment of gender identity and gender role. American Journal of Occupational Therapy 50:535–544

Haboubi N, Lincoln N 2003 Views of health professionals on discussing sexual issues with patients. Disability and Rehabilitation 25:291–296

Herson L, Hart K, Gordon M et al 1999 Identifying and overcoming barriers to providing sexuality information in the clinical setting. Rehabilitation Nursing 24:148–151

Hitchcock J, Wilson H 1992 Personal risking: lesbian self-disclosure of sexual orientation to professional health care providers. Nursing Research 41:178–183

Hodge A 1995 Addressing issue of sexuality with spinal cord injured persons. Orthopaedic Nursing 14(3):21–24

Johns C, Freshwater D 1998 Transforming nursing through reflective practice. Blackwell Science, Oxford

Irwin R 2000 Treatments for patients with sexual problems. Professional Nurse 15:360–364

Jolley S 2002 Taking a sexual history: the role of the nurse. Nursing Times 98(18):39–41

Katz S, Aloni R 1999 Sexual dysfunctions of persons after traumatic brain injury: perceptions of professionals. International Journal of Rehabilitation Research 22:45–53

Laflin M 1996a Sexuality and the elderly. In: Lewis C (ed) Ageing: the health care challenge. FA Davis, Philadelphia

Laflin M 1996b Promoting the sexual health of geriatric patients. Topics in Geriatric Rehabilitation 11(4):43–54

Lemon M 1993 Sexual counselling and spinal cord injury. Sexuality and Disability 11:73–97.

McAlonan S 1996 Improving sexual rehabilitation services: the client's perspective. American Journal of Occupational Therapy 50:826–834

McCann M E 1989 Sexual healing after a heart attack. American Journal of Nursing 89: 1131–1138

Mayers K S, Heller J A 2003 Sexuality and the late stage Huntington's disease patient. Sexuality and Disability 21:91–105

Medlar T, Medlar J 1990 Nursing management of sexuality issues. Journal of Head Trauma Rehabilitation 5:46–61

Meyer-Ruppel A 1999 Incorporating sexuality and the PLISSIT model into your clinical practice. Journal of Gynecologic Oncology Nursing 9:29–31

Miller W 1984 An occupational therapist as a sexual health clinician in the management of spinal cord injuries. Canadian Journal of Occupational Therapy 51:172–175

Mona L R, Krause J S, Norris F H et al 2000 Sexual expression following spinal cord injury. NeuroRehabilitation 15: 121–131

Nolan M, Nolan J 1998 Rehabilitation in multiple sclerosis: the potential nursing contribution. British Journal of Therapy and Rehabilitation 5:370–375

Northcott R, Chard G 2000 Sexual aspects of rehabilitation: the client's perspective. British Journal of Occupational Therapy 63:412–418

Pearson A, Vaughan B, Fitzgerald M 1996 Nursing models for practice, 2nd edn. Butterworth-Heinemann, Oxford

Peate I 2004 Sexuality and sexual health promotion for the older person. British Journal of Nursing 13:188–193

Pope M 1997 Sexual issues for older lesbians and gays. Topics in Geriatric Rehabilitation 12:53–60.

Royal College of Nursing 2000 Sexuality and sexual health in nursing practice. Royal College of Nursing, London

Seidl A, Bullough B, Haughey B et al 1991 Understanding the effects of a myocardial infarction on sexual functioning: a basis for sexual counselling. Rehabilitation Nursing 16:255–264

Shell J, Miller M 1999 The cancer amputee and sexuality. Orthopaedic Nursing 18:53–64

Sherman B 1999 Sex, intimacy and aged care. Jessica Kingsley, London

Shope D 1975 Interpersonal sexuality. WB Saunders, Philadelphia

Smith D 1989 Sexual rehabilitation of the cancer client. Cancer Nursing 12:10–15

Smith D, Babaian R 1992 The effects of treatment for cancer on male fertility and sexuality. Cancer Nursing 15:271–275

Spica M 1989 Sexual counselling standards for the spinal cord-injured. Journal of Neuroscience Nursing 21:56–60

Stuart G, Sundeen S 1979 Principles and practice of psychiatric nursing. C V Mosby, St Louis

Summerville P, McKenna K (1998) Sexuality education and counselling for individuals with a spinal cord injury: implications for occupational therapy, British Journal of Occupational Therapy 61:275–279

Taleporos G, McCabe M P 2002 The impact of sexual esteem, body esteem, and sexual satisfaction on psychological well-being in people with physical disability. Sexuality and Disability 20:177–183

Trombly C 1989 Occupational therapy for physical dysfunction, 2nd edn. Williams & Wilkins, Baltimore

Waterhouse J 1996 Nursing practice related to sexuality: a review and recommendations. Nursing Times Research 1:412–418

White I 2002 Facilitating sexual expression: challenges for contemporary practice. In: Heath H, White I (eds) The challenge of sexuality in health care. Blackwell Science, Oxford

Westgren N, Levi R 1999 Sexuality after injury: interviews with women after traumatic spinal cord injury. Sexuality and Disability 17:309–319

Wilson H, McAndrew S 2000 Sexual health: foundations for practice. Baillière Tindall, London

World Health Organization 1975 Education and treatment in human sexuality: the training of health professionals. WHO Technical Report Series no.572. World Health Organization, Geneva

World Health Organization 2001 International classification of functioning, disability and health. World Health Organization, Geneva

Useful contacts

British Association for Sexual & Relationship Therapy (BASRT)
PO Box 13686

London SW20 9ZH
Tel.: 020 8543 2707
E-mail: info@basrt.org.uk

British Menopause Society
4–6 Eton Place

Marlow
Bucks SL7 2QA
Tel.: 01628 890199

FPA (Formerly the Family Planning Association)
(Information & advice on contraception. SexWare
    catalogue of sexual aids)
2–12 Pentonville Rd
London N1 9FP
Tel.: 020 7837 5432
Helpline: 0845 310 1334
Website: http://www.fpa.org.uk

The Gender Trust
(Offers support to people who are transsexual, gender
    dysphoric or transgenderist)
PO Box 3192
Brighton BN1 3WR
Tel.: 01273 234024
Helpline: 07000 790 347
Website: http://www.gendertrust.org.uk

Institute of Psychosexual Medicine
11 Chandos St
Cavendish Square
London W1G 9DR
Tel.: 020 7580 0631
Website: http://www.ipm.org.uk

London Lesbian & Gay Switchboard
PO Box 7324
London N1 9QS

Tel.: 020 7837 6768
Helpline: 020 7837 7324
Website: http://www.llgs.org.uk

MIND
15–19 Broadway
Stratford
London E15 4BQ
Tel.: 0845 766 0163
Website: http://www.mind.org.uk

RELATE
(Provider of relationship counselling & sex therapy)
11 Little Church St
Rugby CV21 3AW
Tel.: 01788 565675
Website: http://www.relate.org.uk

Sexual Dysfunction Association
Windmill Place Business Centre
2–4 Windmill Lane
Southall
Middlesex UB2 47J
Helpline: 0870 7743571
Website: http://www.sda.uk.net

Sh! Women's Erotic Emporium
57 Hoxton Square
London N1
Tel.: 020 7613 5458
Website: http://www.sh-womenstore.com

Chapter 7

Health Promotion Models

Mary Gottwald

INTRODUCTION

'Health for all' has been on the World Health Organization's agenda for a number of years (Alma Ata Declaration 1978, cited in Katz et al 2002) and is now seen as a challenge for the 21st century. In the UK a number of government policies have been published to facilitate 'health for all', for example *Saving Lives: Our Healthier Nation* (Department of Health 1999), *The NHS Plan* (Department of Health 2000) and National Service Frameworks such as those for Mental Health (Department of Health 1999b), Coronary Heart Disease (Department of Health 2000b) and Older People (Department of Health 2001) and, lastly, *Healthy People 2010*, which aims to promote action and reduce disability (Donatelle 2004).

It is not surprising therefore that the subject of health promotion is topical and relevant to health and social care practitioners working within rehabilitation. The aims of this chapter are:

- To define what is meant by 'health promotion'
- To discuss the relationship between health promotion, rehabilitation and the International Classification of Functioning, Disability and Health (World Health Organization 2001)
- Three models used within health promotion will be outlined and their relationship to rehabilitation discussed, with two case scenarios being used to illustrate the application of each model
- The final section will highlight how models can promote interprofessional working but also lead to barriers to interprofessional working.

CASE STUDY JOEY

Joey is a 50-year-old single unemployed man who lives with his partner on the tenth floor of an apartment block. His partner, John, works as a self-employed plumber. Joey has been unemployed for the last 18 months. He has always enjoyed cooking and now has decided to do all the cooking as it makes him feel that he is contributing to the partnership and therefore increases his self-esteem and makes him less anxious and stressed. However, during his period of unemployment he has put on

4 stone. He has lost motivation to continue with his other hobbies and leads a sedentary lifestyle.

Joey has recently had a heart attack and has been referred to the cardiac rehabilitation pro-gramme. He has not related his heart attack to his increase in weight.

CASE STUDY CHAN

Chan is a 42-year-old man who lives with his wife and two children (aged 10 and 8) in a semi-detached house in a rural community. Following a stroke involving the middle cerebral artery in the non-dominant hemisphere, Chan has been referred to the local rehabilitation unit. Chan has had raised blood pressure for 3 years and has been attending regular appointments with his GP but has not fol-lowed any advice given in relation to his lifestyle.

He reveals to the nurse who is taking his social and medical history that he has smoked 30 ciga-rettes a day since he was 20, mainly when he is at work but also in the evening to help him relax. The rest of his family are healthy but his youngest child has asthma. His job as an accountant is stressful and involves working long hours, which means that he has limited time to spend with his family and friends.

The nurse decides to discuss his smoking. Chan remarks that he would like to stop and says he has done so once before for 3 months but he has started again and now he is disheartened and has a low opinion of himself due to feeling he has failed his family, in particular his daughter who has asthma. Chan has a change in the functions of his left arm and leg. There has been a change in struc-ture in terms of a bleed into the brain.

DEFINING HEALTH PROMOTION

The World Health Organization became an advocate of health promotion over twenty years ago (Thibeault & Hebert 1997) – this was partly due to the recognition of the increase in medical costs and loss of productivity due to unhealthy behaviours (Anderson et al 1999, Thibeault & Hebert 1997). The World Health Organization defines health promotion as:

The process of enabling people to increase control over and improve their health. To reach a state of complete physical, mental and social well being an individual or group must be able to identify and realise aspirations to satisfy needs and to change and cope with the environment.

It is important to note that this definition does not equal 'health educa-tion'. In the past, health education and health promotion are terms that have been used interchangeably. However, health education is a term 'used to describe working with people to give them the knowledge to improve their own health and working towards individual attitude and change' (Ewles & Simnett 2003, p. 24).

Health education is only one aspect of health promotion and tends to focus on the individual, who is held responsible for their behaviour. Health education ignores the wider determinants of health; for example, it ignores the fact that it is not always possible for individuals to make healthy choices. Individuals may not give up smoking because their par-ents and friends smoke or because smoking relieves the stress caused by not having a job/having a pressurised job/having children who behave badly – in other words due to social pressures.

Health promotion is much wider than health education and includes a variety of activities with responsibility being held collectively by society. Those working within rehabilitation can include health promotion activities within their roles and effectively promote health on either a one-to-one basis or a group basis. It must also be remembered that, following government initiatives, whole populations can also be targeted (Ewles & Simnett 2003, Bennett & Murphy 1997).

Activities include *preventative health services*, for example, screening for disease and immunisation. *Health education programmes* include highlighting the dangers of smoking or excessive alcohol intake, the benefits of a healthy diet or the benefits of taking exercise. *Community-based work* will involve health and social care professionals assisting communities to take collective action in order to identify and meet their own health needs. *Public health policy* ensures that having good health is not solely the individual's responsibility but also the responsibility of the government and local and national health departments. *Environmental health policies* ensure that the focus is on improving amenities such as safe water, including fluoride in water to reduce tooth decay, or reducing air pollution. *Organisational development* might involve an organisation such as a hospital ensuring that its policies promote the health of all employees by having healthy menus in the canteen. The final activity suggested involves *Economic and regulatory activities*, which could relate to policy such as raising taxes on alcohol to reduce alcoholism (Ewles & Simnett 2003, p. 28).

Although the above activities demonstrate the breadth of health promotion work, not all these aspects will be part of each health promoter's role.

HEALTH PROMOTION AND REHABILITATION

One question health- and social-care professionals who work within rehabilitation can ask themselves is: How does health promotion fit within their remit? Barnes & Ward (2000) define rehabilitation as 'an active and dynamic process by which a disabled person is helped to acquire knowledge and skills in order to maximise physical, psychological and social function; it is a process that maximises functional ability' (p. 4).

By comparing this to the definition provided by the World Health Organization, similarities can be seen. For example, both health promotion and rehabilitation are concerned with developing skills and changing the social environment in order to improve health and functional ability. Both rehabilitation and health promotion focus on all aspects that are pertinent to the person. It is evident, therefore, that those health and social care practitioners who work within rehabilitation could include some of the health promotion activities identified by Ewles & Simnett (2003) within their current roles. Practitioners would aim to **empower** the clients they work with to **achieve behavioural change** – this being the main aim of health promotion work.

The International Classification of Functioning, Disability and Health (World Health Organization 2001) provides a scientific basis for understanding and studying health and can also be used as part of the framework to identify the focus of interventions, which in turn will facilitate necessary behavioural changes within the health promotion aspects of a person's rehabilitation programme.

CASE STUDY JOEY

Impairment	Activity Limitations	Participation Restriction
• Anxiety	• Difficulties with instrumental activities of daily living	• Unable to carry out domestic tasks
• Stress		• Unable to participate in leisure activities
• Reduced self-esteem		

CASE STUDY CHAN

Impairment	Activity Limitations	Participation Restriction
• High muscle tone	• Difficulty with activities of daily living	• Unable to carry out roles related to job
• Reduced sensation	• Difficulty with fine hand coordination tasks	• Unable to participate in family activities
• Abnormal reflex activity	• Difficulties with work tasks	
• Reduced voluntary movements		
• Stress		

If part of the rehabilitation focus is on developing Joey and Chan's self-esteem and self-efficacy and reducing anxiety and stress levels, then this should facilitate behavioural changes in relation to healthier eating and reduction/cessation of smoking, i.e. the health promotion component of their rehabilitation programmes. If behavioural changes are successful then the likelihood of further heart attacks or strokes is diminished.

MODELS OF HEALTH PROMOTION

There are a number of models that could be used within health promotion, however, for the purpose of this chapter three models will be outlined and then their relationship to rehabilitation discussed. These models are: the Stages of Change Model (Prochaska & Di Clemente 1982), Beattie's model (1991, cited in Naidoo & Wills 2000) and the Health Action Model (Tones 1987, cited in Tones & Tilford 2001). Examples of other models that would work equally well within rehabilitation are the Health Belief Model (Hochbaum 1958, cited in Tones & Green 2004), the Theory of Reasoned Action (Fishbein & Ajzen 1975, cited in Naidoo & Wills 2000) and the Health Promotion Model (Pender et al 2002). A case study will be used to illustrate how each model can be used within rehabilitation.

Models are used within health promotion work as they provide health and social care practitioners with a clear framework that first of all helps them to understand multifaceted situations, then aids their decision-making and enables them to plan effective intervention with their clients. They are a way of linking ideas together as well as showing the relationship between theory and practice (Ewles & Simnett 2003, Naidoo & Wills 1998, 2000). Evidence has indicated that models are open to criticism; for example, Anderson et al (1999) highlight issues from research carried out applying the Stages of Change Model proposed by Prochaska & Di Clemente (1982). Although evidence suggests the Stages of Change Model can reliably and validly be used by clinicians, no strategies are suggested that will help the health and social care practititioner to move their client from one stage to the next.

By being aware of a number of models that can be used to promote health within rehabilitation programmes, health and social care practitioners can choose the most appropriate model to use as the framework for intervention. Choice of model may also depend on the client's culture, socioeconomic status and personal values and beliefs. However, it is suggested that these models could be used within a variety of rehabilitation settings, e.g. within mental health and physical disability services.

The first model chosen is what is known as a descriptive model and the latter two are analytical models. 'Descriptive models identify the diversity of existing practice but make no judgements about which kind of practice is preferable. Analytical models are explicit about the values underpinning practice and often prioritise certain kinds of practice over others' (Naidoo & Wills 2001, p. 292).

STAGES OF CHANGE MODEL (PROCHASKA & DI CLEMENTE 1982)

This model can be used to enable health and social care professionals working within rehabilitation and their clients to work alongside each other. Evidence suggests that this model can be used widely. For example, it has been used with people who have addictive behaviours such as smoking and alcoholism (Prochaska et al 1992, Otake & Shimai 2001, Mendel & Hipkins 2002), with those with mental health issues and co-occurring disorders (Finnell 2003) and those who have a chronic illness, for example asthma or diabetes (Cassidy 1999, Natarajan et al 2002, Vallis et al 2003). Hilton et al (1999) have used the model to promote behavioural change in those at risk of coronary heart disease.

Prochaska & Di Clemente (1982) described this process model both as a linear and circular model and maintained that individuals go through a number of stages in order to change their behaviour. In the linear model, the clients that health and social care professionals work with would progress from one stage to the next before successfully achieving improved health behaviours. The linear model does not allow for relapses (Anderson et al 1999).

However, Prochaska & Di Clemente recognise the difficulties attaining successful behavioural change and stressed that some individuals may need to go through the process more than once – hence the cyclical model. According to Prochaska & Di Clemente, those who want to give up smoking need to go round the cycle on average three times before succeeding. Some may go around the cycle a number of times and then make the decision that they will continue to smoke as they 'do not like continued failure . . . and try to resume the life of a satisfied smoker' (p. 284). In this case, the person's autonomy must be respected.

There are five stages to this model (Fig. 7.1):

1. Pre-contemplation stage
2. Contemplation stage
3. Commitment stage
4. Action stage/Maintenance
5. Relapse.

Readers should note that literature uses different terminologies for the third stage. Prochaska & DiClemente (1982) use 'determination', Prochaska et al (1992) and Anderson et al (1999) use 'preparation' and Ewles & Simnett (2003) 'commitment'.

During the first three stages health and social care practitioners work alongside clients, preparing them for change. Motivation is the key to successful behavioural change, so once clients believe that their expectations will be met and that change can take place, they will 'commit' themselves to the health promotion programme.

Motivational interviewing may be a useful technique to include as part of the rehabilitation and health promotion programme, and has been used with those who have mental health disorders, diabetes and HIV, as it is thought to increase insight and compliance with interventions (Rusch & Corrigan 2002). Motivational interviewing 'allows the person to explore and discover the advantages and disadvantages of their behaviours for themselves' (Rusch & Corrigan 2002, p. 28). Realistic goals also need to be determined and a caring relationship that includes trust is essential between practitioners and clients (Prochaska & Di Clemente 1982). If goals set are SMART (specific, measurable, achievable, realistic and with a timescale) and if goals are set by the practitioner and client together, then it can make achievement of goals more successful.

First, it is important to note that some individuals may decide not to change even though they have been given information about the benefits of, for instance, giving up smoking, losing weight, drinking less alcohol. They may also make the decision that they are unable to change.

Second, individuals may decide to exit at any stage of this model and some individuals may remain in one stage for some time; for example, those with obsessive–compulsive disorder may remain in the 'contemplation stage', as they are continually seeking information in the hope that their issues will suddenly be resolved without them having to go through the 'action stage' (Prochaska & Di Clemente 1982).

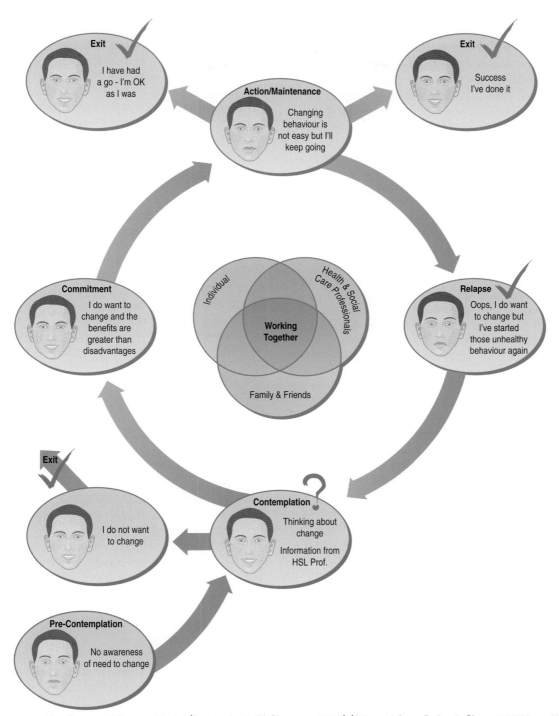

Figure 7.1   The Stages of Change Model (Prochaska & Di Clemente 1982) (Adapted from Ewles & Simnett 2003, p. 274)

CASE STUDY JOEY

Pre-contemplation stage

Someone who denies that there is a problem, or is not aware of the consequences and does not recognise that there is a need to change their health related behaviour, will not progress beyond this stage until they make the decision that they want to change their behaviour (Prochaska & Di Clemente 1982, Ewles & Simnett 2003). At this point, the individual may only see the 'costs' to them and cannot see any benefits from changing their behaviour (Rusch & Corrigan 2002).

Joey has identified that he has been stressed and anxious; therefore, initially, rehabilitation could focus on coping strategies to reduce his stress and anxiety (Anderson et al 1999).

In the pre-contemplation stage, health education, as part of the rehabilitation programme, is also appropriate. Information and advice may be given to raise Joey's awareness about the risks related to his health related behaviour. This information will enable Joey to make a decision as to whether to continue with his present diet and sedentary lifestyle. At this stage it would not be helpful to tell Joey to eat a more healthy diet and lose weight. Advice given could be general, for example, letting him know that there is help available from a dietitian. Giving the person the opportunity to go away and reflect on the advice is essential. However, assumptions should not be made that, just because Joey has been given appropriate information, this will not necessarily lead to weight reduction – all other factors need to be considered. It is for this reason that the issues behind Joey's stress and anxiety need to be considered (McDougall 2001).

Activities that would motivate Joey to change his unhealthy lifestyle, i.e. lose weight, could also be included in the rehabilitation programme.

Contemplation stage

Having attended the cardiac rehabilitation programme Joey is now more aware of the risks related to his unhealthy behaviour and may be thinking about changing. However, although he may begin to see the benefits of changing his behaviour, he still feels that the costs outweigh the benefits (Rusch & Corrigan 2002).

Increasing Joey's self-empowerment is important and therefore advice can be more specific – healthy versus non-healthy diets; the effects of an unhealthy diet on the heart. Sessions on healthy eating could be included in the cardiac rehabilitation programme. By including these sessions in the rehabilitation programme Joey would not be the main focus of the session, as this information would also be appropriate for other group participants.

Health and social care professionals must not assume that, just because Joey is aware of the risks related to his behaviour, i.e. the consequences, he will be able to select the best strategies to achieve weight loss.

Commitment stage

Once Joey has been provided with accurate information and has been made aware of alternative choices, strategies to help with decision-making can be given. Joey can make the decision to change and then can be referred to a dietitian, who would help him plan a specific diet. It is only at this point that Joey will be able to see that the benefits of changing his behaviour are greater than the costs (Rusch & Corrigan 2002).

Action stage/Maintenance stages

As part of his rehabilitation programme, Joey begins to change his diet and monitor his weight; in other words, he begins to practise new behaviours. Behaviour change strategies are still needed and continuing advice and support about changing routines could be helpful.

At this point Joey may exit the cycle. However, as previously mentioned, this is not a simple process and may take 6 months or more (Rusch & Corrigan 2002). If a further life event occurs that increases his anxiety and stress levels and once again lowers his self-esteem, Joey may return to his previous unhealthy eating habits and thus the relapse stage may be entered. Unless Joey finds employment he may revert back to his 'comfort eating'. It is important that this is not seen as failure but as a normal part of the process. It is essential for encouragement to continue, which will empower Joey to make the decision to enter the contemplation stage again.

CASE STUDY CHAN

Anderson et al (1999) state that the model that has been used most frequently with people who smoke is the Stages of Change Model. According to Prochaska & Di Clemente (1982), individuals remain in each stage for different periods of time. It is important for health and social care practitioners not to make assumptions and to be aware of varying timeframes. The individual needs to feel ready to move on to the next stage and should not move on just because the practitioner deems them to be ready. If they do not want to move on then it must not be assumed that they are being resistive to change.

According to Prochaska & Di Clemente (1982), Anderson et al (1999) and McDougall (2001), smokers may remain in the contemplation stage for 2 weeks or any time up to 1 year. They may remain in the commitment stage for between 2 hours and 2 months, while the maintenance/action stage may take longer and last between 6 and 12 months. The first 3–6 months are the most difficult and a time when relapse may occur. The next 6–12 months are less difficult but strategies need to be continued to ensure successful behavioural change in relation to giving up smoking.

Chan has successfully stopped smoking before and therefore at the time of his visit to the rehabilitation unit he is in the relapse stage of the Stages of Change Model. As he has been successful before, health promotion advice could begin by ascertaining what strategies worked for Chan before and what made him start smoking again. Health and social care practitioners could begin to help Chan identify the cause of his stress and identify how strong Chan's commitment was the first time he decided to give up smoking. They also need to consider Chan's levels of self-efficacy. The more able Chan believes himself to be in dealing with the internal and external pressures to smoke, the more likely he is to succeed this time with giving up smoking.

As Chan has remarked that he would like to stop smoking again (contemplation stage), practitioners could begin with offering advice to help him stop smoking again (commitment stage). He could be offered support as an individual at an outpatient's clinic, if this was appropriate, or in a 'stop smoking' group, which runs in his local health centre. Support from family and friends is essential and consideration needs to be given to the issue that friends may smoke and therefore add more pressure. Finally what is important this time around the cycle is that Chan needs to value the consequences of his behavioural change.

One of the criticisms of using this model with Chan is that the focus is on 'giving up smoking'. The model does not really focus on the reasons why Chan has started smoking again, for example, his stressful job that involves working long hours and therefore gives him limited time for socialising with his family and friends. However, these factors could be taken into account as part of his rehabilitation programme following his stroke. We can therefore see how this health promotion model can be used within Chan's rehabilitation programme.

BEATTIE'S MODEL (1991)

There appears to be limited research published in relation to Beattie's model but it is still deemed to be useful for helping practitioners analyse current strategies used within the rehabilitation team. It could help the team to make changes that promote client-centred practice and encourages the team to increase their self-awareness and question their own values and assumptions. This would enable the team to change from using a very top-down approach to a more bottom-up approach. Having said this, each quadrant is valuable.

This model gives the health and social care practitioner a choice of two modes of intervention and four approaches to choose from to help them plan and organise their health promotion activities with either the individual or the community. Each quadrant suggests different approaches and a variety of health promotion activities that could be carried out as part of a rehabilitation programme (Naidoo & Wills 1998, 2000, 2001, Kerr 2002) (Fig. 7.2).

The authoritative mode of intervention is considered to be a top-down approach, i.e. the person/community is 'told what to do' and are encouraged to change their behaviours to those suggested by health and social care professionals, whereas the negotiated mode is seen as a bottom-up approach where the person/community identify their own health needs and then professionals work with them to agree what the best course of action is.

One issue for practitioners to consider is the mode of intervention currently used within practice. If the top-down approach has been the main mode of intervention then practitioners could use this model to analyse their practice. The model may highlight a need for potential change, which may result in practitioners using the bottom-up, more client-centred mode of intervention.

Figure 7.2   Beattie's model (Adapted with permission from Naidoo & Wills 2001, p. 295)

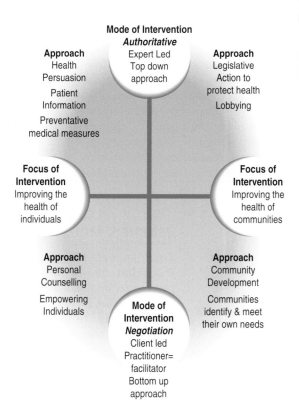

CASE STUDY JOEY

First of all the rehabilitation team would need to select which quadrant is pertinent. If clients have no idea that there is a need to change their health-related behaviours, initially the authoritative/individual quadrant may be used. Then once the client is aware and decides to change their health-related behaviours, the negotiated/individual quadrant may be identified as being the most appropriate.

Mode of intervention – authoritative/focus of intervention – the individual

In this quadrant the focus is on the individual to change their behaviour. The professionals lead the interventions; for example, the dietitian may provide Joey with information on losing weight following his cardiac arrest – the advice is deemed to be important by the dietitian rather than Joey. Other health and social care practitioners would identify to Joey that his participation in an exercise programme as part of the cardiac rehabilitation programme would be important.

Mode of intervention – negotiated/focus of intervention – the individual

Following his heart attack Joey makes the decision to go on a diet. In this mode, he leads the intervention. Joey decides that he wants to discuss his diet and initiates the sessions with a member of staff from the cardiac rehabilitation programme, who then acts as the facilitator. If Joey asks for information on healthier eating, then the practitioner can provide him with this.

Losing weight may add to Joey's levels of stress and anxiety and therefore he may also ask for support while he is on his diet, i.e. counselling. At the same time, if the rehabilitation team are working with Joey to improve his self-esteem and self-efficacy, he is more likely to feel empowered to follow the dietitians advice.

Mode of intervention – authoritative/focus of intervention – the community

In this quadrant professionals aim to protect the community by improving the community's health.

They may, for example, work with community members and campaign to improve food-labelling regulations, lead legislative action and lobby the government to make changes.

Community initiatives that foster local weight-management support groups and develop health-related services such as cardiac care support groups could also be developed. Following the National Service Framework for coronary care, the agenda for these initiatives is primarily authoritative, as the government and not the community has identified the agenda. However, the focus is on improving the health of the community, of which Joey is a member.

In order for Joey to understand the food labels, and therefore which foods are healthier, the rehabilitation team may revert to the first quadrant discussed above and provide information on content and nutritional value of food that would help Joey to make choices that will help him to lose weight.

Mode of intervention – negotiated / focus of intervention – the community

Community development seeks to empower the community to meet their own needs, for example, Joey may identify that the community in which he lives has a need for more fresh fruit and vegetables to be sold at the local community shop. Health professionals from the cardiac rehabilitation programme and community members may liaise with local authority councillors who in turn may enhance the community's skills and empower them to be able to negotiate with the owner of the shop. This would also make it easier for Joey to walk to the local shop and buy more healthy food.

The cardiac rehabilitation group could be encouraged to plan healthier menus together, thus taking some of the responsibility from the individual. As an individual, Joey could then make an informed choice and decide to cook healthier meals for himself and his partner.

THE HEALTH ACTION MODEL (TONES 1987)

This model (Fig. 7.3) initially presented by Tones in the 1970s (Tones & Green 2004) initially appears complex and does not look at whether people are ready to change, like Prochaska and Di Clemente's 'Stages of Change Model'. However, it is useful in that it can be used to analyse whether a health promotion activity is likely to have any impact on the person's intentions, leading them to change their behaviour.

First, this model focuses on three belief systems – the normative (social pressures), motivation and belief system (Fig. 7.3). These systems influence whether an individual is likely to change their health related behaviour. For example, if the social environment is not suitable or if the individual does not have the necessary knowledge and skills, then the individual may not be able to change their behaviour.

Second, this model emphasises the importance of personality dimension (self-sentiment and self-concept) on behavioural intention. It presumes that a person with high self-esteem, an internal locus of control and a positive self-concept will be more likely to perform positive health-related behaviours. On the other hand, a person with low self-esteem and an external locus of control may feel that they are not able to perform positive health-related behaviours for reasons beyond their control (Tones & Tilford 2001, Katz et al 2002, Ewles & Simnett 2003).

The model therefore emphasises the importance of empowerment and facilitation of positive health behaviours through the development of a

Figure 7.3 The Health Action Model (Reproduced with the permission of Nelson Thornes Ltd from *Health Promotion: Effectiveness, efficiency and equity*, ISBN 0 7487 4527 0 – Keith Tones and Sylvia Tilford (Tones & Tilford 2001), first published in 1990)

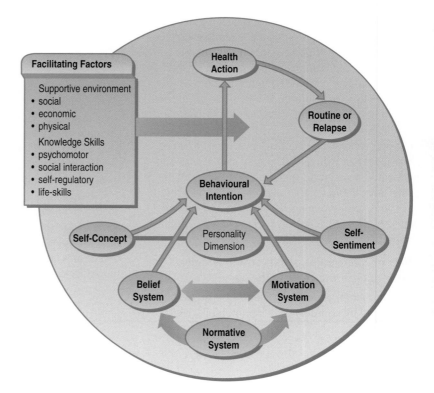

person's self-esteem, self-concept and 'life skills'. Health and social care professionals can work with the individual, and/or at a national/local level, to address the basic environmental determinants of health (Ewles & Simnett 2003, p. 272). They also have a responsibility to work with the individual to identify their values and beliefs and the particulars that lead to negative health-related behaviours in order to ensure that individuals routinely include healthy behavioural activities within their lifestyles (Tones & Green 2004).

As with the Stages of Change Model, it can be seen that, even though the model can be used as a framework within rehabilitation, relapses may occur. In this instance it is important for the rehabilitation professional to re-evaluate how the three belief systems can be used and to continue to work with individuals to develop their knowledge, skills, self-concept and self-sentiment further so that they can feel empowered to make behavioural changes that become part of their daily routine.

CASE STUDY JOEY

If the health and social care professional uses this model, then part of the rehabilitation programme would include developing Joey's assertiveness skills and would include activities to develop his self-esteem. The latter part of the programme could include work rehabilitation in order to develop his skills further. If this led to paid employment or voluntary work then it is likely his self-esteem would be improved and therefore Joey would value himself more. He would then hopefully be able to maintain a healthy weight, reducing the likelihood of a further heart attack. However, if Joey is unsuccessful in finding employment and if local policy does not encourage healthy eating choices then it is less likely that Joey will achieve behavioural changes.

CASE STUDY CHAN

Chan has identified that he wants to give up smoking and spend more time with his family. Alongside his rehabilitation programme, he has been attending the local support group, which is facilitated by a health and social care professional. The focus of this model would differ from that of Prochaska & Di Clemente's model. Here the professional works alongside Chan and other members of the group to develop their knowledge of the harmful effects of smoking. The professional would aim to improve Chan's self-esteem, and skills in assertiveness can also be taught, which would enable Chan to review his roles at work, thus reducing the pressure of long working hours. In other words, the reasons behind Chan's smoking are explored, in the belief that dealing with these problems would enable Chan to give up smoking permanently.

The Health Action Model stresses the importance of Chan's self-concept in facilitating change. The model also suggests that working with others (the support group) can help and emphasises that barriers can prevent change – the pressures of working long hours may have led to Chan feeling stressed and his subsequent continuation of unhealthy related behaviours. The model does not simply focus on Chan's behavioural intention but considers the wider implications, knowledge and skills needed to achieve the desired healthy behaviour.

HEALTH PROMOTION MODELS AND INTER–PROFESSIONAL WORKING

In today's client-centred practice arena it is essential for health and social care practitioners working in public and private sector organizations to collaborate and work together with each other as well as their clients.

Practitioners are governed by a number of government policies and directives and therefore, through collaboration, those working in different agencies and services can ensure that practice is more clearly coordinated, which in turn can only improve the seamless service, quality and continuity of care provided for clients and carers (Barr 1997, Proctor-Childs et al 1998, Payne 2000).

By working together and using a health promotion model as one of the frameworks for practice, interprofessional teams will be able to plan, monitor and evaluate their practice more easily and will be working 'with rather than alongside each other' (Proctor-Childs et al 1998, p. 616), and therefore any potential conflict can be avoided. The models described could encourage practitioners to reflect on practice, examine their values and beliefs and possibly change from using top-down approaches to bottom-up approaches, enabling a greater sense of client empowerment and client-led service.

Models of health promotion can unify practice but do not prevent different professionals from carrying out discipline-specific interventions. Models can ensure that each professional is guided by activities in each stage of the Stages of Change Model or each quadrant of Beattie's Model.

On the other hand, confusion and conflict could occur between team members and/or between health and social care professionals and clients if there is no agreement on the best approach to intervention. For instance, clients may wish to continue their unhealthy behaviours (smoking, excessive eating), whereas professionals could deem that these behaviours should change in order to prevent further strokes or heart attacks. In this case, professionals can support each other and their clients who decide to revert back to unhealthy related behaviours, while continuing with other rehabilitation services offered.

In interprofessional working it is essential to identify goals that are responsive to both the client and their carers. If there is no consensus on which health promotion model to use, goals set may be unclear for both the professional and client and therefore a breakdown in communication and collaboration could occur (Mariano 1992, Lindeke & Block 1998).

It is therefore essential for the rehabilitation team to select the most appropriate health promotion model to use within their programmes.

CONCLUSION

Three models used within health promotion work have been outlined; however, it is important for health and social care professionals working within rehabilitation to keep an open mind. These models can help practitioners to plan their rehabilitation programmes but do not have to be used prescriptively and perhaps thought can be given to using a mixture of models at the same time, or perhaps one model might initially be used as the framework and then, as clients achieve their goals/change their goals, the professional can use another model as the framework.

It is also essential to keep in mind clients' views about causes and prevention of ill health and, as mentioned in the Health Action Model, the extent to which clients feel they can change their lives; their sociocultural and religious beliefs; whether they want to change – and, as discussed in the Stages of Change Model, whether the benefits outweigh the disadvantages.

Lastly, as well as remembering the individual factors (empowering clients, developing skills, enhancing self-esteem), it is important to remember the environmental and social factors – if the latter two do not facilitate the most healthy choices then it will be difficult to achieve behavioural changes resulting in improved health.

QUESTIONS FOR DISCUSSION

- How do you decide which health promotion model to use?
- How do you decide whether to use one health promotion model or a mixture of models?
- As a team, how will the client's views about causes and prevention of ill health be considered?
- How will you ensure that the individual, environmental and social factors will be considered for each person referred to you for rehabilitation?

References

Anderson S, Keller C, McGowan N 1999 Smoking cessation: the state of the science. The utility of the transtheoretical model in guiding interventions in smoking cessation. Online Journal of Knowledge Synthesis for Nursing 6(9)

Barnes M, Ward A 2000 Textbook of rehabilitation medicine. Oxford University Press, Oxford

Barr O 1997 Interdisciplinary teamwork: consideration of the challenges. British Journal of Nursing 6:1005–1010

Beattie A 1991 knowledge and control in health promotion: a test case for social policy and social theory. In Gabe J. Calhan M, Bury M (eds) the sociology of the health service. Routledge: London.

Bennett P, Murphy S 1997 Psychology and health promotion. Open University Press, Buckingham

Cassidy C 1999 Using the transtheoretical model to facilitate behavior change in patients with chronic illness. Journal of American Academic Nursing Practice 11:281–287

Department of Health 1999a Saving lives: our healthier nation. HMSO, London

Department of Health 1999b Mental health: national service frameworks. HMSO, London

Department of Health 2000a The NHS plan: a plan for investment, a plan for reform. HMSO, Norwich

Department of Health 2000b Coronary heart disease: national service frameworks. HMSO, London

Department of Health 2001 Older people: national service frameworks. HMSO, London

Donatelle R 2004 Access to health. Pearson Education, London

Ewles L, Simnett I 2003 Promoting health: a practical guide, 5th edn. Baillière Tindall, London

Finnell D 2003 Addictions services. Use of the transtheoretical model for individuals with co-occurring disorders. Community Mental Health Journal 39:3–15

Hilton S, Doherty S, Kendrick T et al 1999 Promotion of healthy behaviour among adults at increased risk of coronary heart disease in general practice: methodology and baseline data from the Change of Heart study. Health Education Journal 58:3–16

Hochbaum, GM 1958 Public participation in medical screening programs: A socio psychological study. US Government printing office: Washington DC.

Katz J, Peberdy A, Douglas J 2002 Promoting health: knowledge and practice. Macmillan, Basingstoke

Kerr J 2002 Community health promotion: challenges for practice. Elsevier, London

Lindeke L, Block D 1998 Maintaining professional integrity in the midst of interdisciplinary collaboration. Nursing Outlook 46:213–218

Mariano C 1992 Interdisciplinary collaboration a practice imperative Healthcare Trends and Transition 5:10–12, 24–25

McDougall P 2001 Changing behaviour: models in health promotion. Community Practitioner 74:302–304

Mendel E, Hipkins J 2002 Motivating learning disabled offenders with alcohol-related problems: a pilot study. British Journal of Learning Disabilities 30:153–158

Naidoo J, Wills J 1998 Practising health promotion: dilemmas and challenges. Baillière Tindall, London

Naidoo J, Wills, J. 2000 Health promotion: foundations for practice, 2nd edn. Baillière Tindall, London

Naidoo J, Wills J 2001 Health studies: an introduction. Palgrave, Basingstoke

Natarajan S, Clyburn E, Brown R 2002 Association of exercise stages of change with glycemic control in individuals with type 2 diabetes. American Journal of Health Promotion 17:72–75

Otake K, Shimai S 2001 Adopting the stage model for smoking acquisition in Japanese adolescents. Journal of Health Psychology 6:629–643

Payne M 2000 Teamwork in multiprofessional care. Palgrave, Basingstoke

Pender N, Murdaugh C, Parsons MA. 2002 Health promotion in nursing practice. Prentice Hall, Englewood Cliffs, NJ

Prochaska J, Di Clemente C 1982 Transtheoretical therapy: towards a more integrative model of change. Psychotherapy: Theory, Research and Practice 19:276–288

Prochaska J, Di Clemente C, Norcross J 1992 In search of how people change. American Psychologist 47:1102–1114

Proctor-Childs T, Freeman M, Miller C 1998 Visions of teamwork: the realities of an interdisciplinary approach. British Journal of Therapy and Rehabilitation 5:616–635

Rusch N, Corrigan P 2002 Motivational interviewing to improve insight and treatment adherence in schizophrenia. Psychiatric Rehabilitation Journal 26:23–32

Thibeault R, Hebert M 1997 A congruent model for health promotion in occupational therapy. Occupational Therapy International 4:271–293

Tones BK 1987 Devising strategies for preventing drug misuse: the role of the health action model. Health education research, 2, 305–318

Tones K, Tilford S 2001 Health promotion: effectiveness, efficiency and equity, 3rd edn. Nelson Thornes, Cheltenham

Tones K, Green J 2004 Health promotion, planning and strategies. Sage Publications, London

Vallis M, Ruggiero L, Greene G et al 2003 Stages of change for healthy eating in diabetes. Diabetes Care 26:1468–1474

World Health Organization 2001 International classification of functioning, disability and health. World Health Organization, Geneva. Available on-line at: http://www.who.int/icf/icftemplate.cfm

Chapter **8**

The *Kawa* (River) Model:
Client centred rehabilitation in cultural context
Michael K. Iwama

INTRODUCTION

Culture in rehabilitation is often regarded as an individual client matter rather than a fundamental, central and pervasive element of rehabilitation philosophy, theory and practice. Contemporary approaches in rehabilitation are heavily influenced by Western cultural contexts from which they were developed, and hence may not be as appropriate for clients and professionals situated outside mainstream Western cultural norms. The aim of this chapter is to illuminate the cultural aspects of rehabilitation theory through an occupational therapy conceptual model developed outside the Western world.

The *Kawa*/River model is presented with the aims of:

- Demonstrating the relationship between cultural context and the structure and concepts of conceptual models in rehabilitation
- Challenging rehabilitation professionals to examine the cultural boundaries of their own approaches
- Discussing the implications of cultural relevance to client-centred rehabilitation practice.

The International Classification of Functioning, Disability and Health (ICF; World Health Organization 2001) represents an important development toward acknowledging the wider social complexities and contexts associated with people's health and health related states. In rehabilitation theory and practice, matters of disability that were once conceptualised predominantly from a medical-pathology perspective, are now appreciated more broadly. In the new ICF framework social and environmental factors are accorded greater emphasis, leading to a more inclusive and less pathology- and impairment-centred view of health and disability. The framework has continued to advance rehabilitation toward more holistic, bio-psycho-social perspectives (World Health Organization 2001, p. 9) and shows promise in bringing client-centred care in practice much closer to realisation. A universal framework like the ICF may equitably classify individuals' states of health and disability and guide rehabilitation toward a more consistent and potentially better quality of rehabilitative care.

Though the ICF continues to show promise in bringing about a more universal and systematic approach to classifying and thus shaping approaches to issues of disability and health, there are gaps appearing in the interim. Arguably one of the larger challenges to the utility of the ICF or any universal classification system based on Western health practices and norms is 'culture' and the diverse ways in which individuals and communities view and experience their worlds and construct their particular understandings of health and disability. The universality (World Health Organization 2001, p. 14) purported in authoritative classification systems and their aims to systematically explain and guide matters of health and disability for all can potentially fall short of adequately explaining the rehabilitative health needs of individuals and societies who find themselves situated on and outside the margins of its categories. In other words, from a cultural perspective, the varying social experiences in varying contexts of health and disability, and alternate perspectives of health that transcend the individual level, may require some flexibility and accommodation in our current theoretical frameworks. Consideration of alternate culturally relevant theory and knowledge systems might be helpful in augmenting or complementing the ICF framework.

Most contemporary conceptual models of rehabilitation have been raised out of Western social and cultural contexts and reflect the characteristics and features germane to Western interpretations and views of reality. This includes health and, in the field of rehabilitation, what is worth doing and what constitutes a state of wellness to which rehabilitation professionals endeavour to restore their clients. In particular, most contemporary models in rehabilitation construe the individual to be central to and agent in a surrounding but distinctly separate social, physical, economic and political environment. For those who do not abide in this particular 'normal' experience of daily Western life nor fit neatly into the categories set forth by a particular health model, current theory and practices may be inadequate and even exclusive in some instances. For example, the practice of locating disability in the individual constructing it as a personal tragedy rather than a societal one, with the mandate to enhance independence and autonomy, may be poorly comprehended and even maladaptive for those who view the world and situate matters of wellbeing in a less rational, more naturalistic and social collective oriented way.

Western ideologies and influences, which have shaped theoretical and epistemological discourse and practices in rehabilitation over the past decades, are being recognised increasingly within a wider and more diverse global context. This is becoming clearer as rehabilitation professionals increasingly encounter challenges in carrying out their therapeutic mandates with people from differing and varied cultural origins. There may be a tendency to situate the problem of incongruence on the client, often construing the problem to be one of compromised communication or client 'noncompliance', rather than the cultural norms and imperatives embedded in the rehabilitation programme's philosophy and mandate. Rehabilitation professionals may need to examine the tacit philosophy and mandates of their own professions to determine how they resonate and agree with their clients' cultural values and norms around health and wellbeing. Cultural competence in rehabilitative care should go beyond merely understanding and being sensitive to the cultural features of the client. Cultural competence should also include an understanding of the cultural nature of one's own health profession (Iwama 2003). Rehabilitation mandates and the classification systems they employ may need to be scrutinised and thoughtfully considered from the client perspective as health professionals and policy makers endeavour to guide and manage the care of populations.

If we allow a broader definition of culture that transcends race and ethnicity and recognise it as shared experiences giving rise to common meanings and understandings of phenomena and objects around us, then we can begin to appreciate that each of our health disciplines that make up an interdisciplinary approach possesses its own culturally and contextually bound ideology, structure, content and approaches. In this way, rehabilitation professions, such as medicine or occupational therapy, can be also viewed as having a particular culture. Each possesses, in their worlds, a shared specialised language, tacit rules of conduct in carrying out its activities, established social practices that follow a pattern that help to identify its members from other professionals, and certain institutional conditions of knowledge production (Smith 2000) that help to unify its discourse. Critical examination of the theory of most health professions will reveal that their existing conceptual models are culturally situated and that their specificity can often, despite best intentions, unwittingly exclude both clients and therapists who abide in differing cultural contexts that sit outside of a standard or universally viewed norm.

Recognising the challenges that culture presents to the discourse on rehabilitation theory and universal classification systems lends some support to the need for culturally relevant models. New models may need to stray from any tendency to impose explanatory frameworks of health on to populations out of cultural context. If rehabilitation is to achieve its aims of minimising the effects of disability and enabling people to resume better health states in a proper cultural context, not only might the forms of practice need to undergo change but also the theoretical frameworks and knowledge systems that drive and inform them.

In this chapter, such a new model originating from an East Asian occupational therapy setting is introduced. What is presented here is not necessarily a new, competing model of rehabilitation practice but rather an example of how cultural views of reality and wellbeing are tied to and expressed in theoretical material constructed in a particular context. The *Kawa* Model shows a culturally specific way in which disability and healthy states are considered in a particular dynamic between people and the contexts in which they live. Such a strikingly different conceptual model not only portrays how certain non-Western people can view matters of wellbeing and disability but may aid Western rehabilitation professionals to view the cultural features and biases within their own conceptual frameworks and classification systems. A conceptual model based on differing ontology supported by Eastern ways of knowing offers an alternate perch from which to view and make sense of our conventional approaches founded and refined in explanations of Western social experience.

Ultimately, the models and theoretical frameworks employed by rehabilitation professionals to make sense of their clients' worlds of health and disability and to guide effective and meaningful interventions, should resonate with their clients' views and explanations of the same.

BEYOND INDIVIDUALISM AND SELF-DETERMINISM: EMERGING REHABILITATION IMPERATIVES

Self in relation to environs: a context for health and wellbeing

Culture can be appreciated at the core of most contemporary conceptual models of rehabilitation and is particularly observable in how the 'self' is socially constructed and situated in relation to the surrounding environment (context). The interpretations and meanings we derive through what we do in the world may vary according to how this dualism is regarded and understood. The self, in Western social depictions, as evident in current occupational therapy conceptual models such as the Model of Human Occupation (Kielhofner 2002) and the Canadian Model of Occupational Performance (Canadian Association of Occupational Therapists 2003), construe the self as being not only centrally and focally situated in the centre of the universe but also understood to be rationally separate and superior in power and status to the environment and nature. Wellbeing is constructed to be contingent on the extent to which the *self* can act on and demonstrate its ability to control one's perceived circumstances located in the environment. Failure or compromise in controlling the environment is construed in such terms as dysfunction and disability. These terms are often pejorative because the self is seen to be falling short of the norm – to be competent, effective and in control. In these world views, dependency can often represent an undesirable state. Dependency is often connoted with disability.

With this particular self-agency comes a sense of entitlement to doing in the present (here and now) that extends temporally into the future (hence a propensity to set goals). It is not uncommon in many Western experiences for people to strive to control their immediate circumstances and to set future objectives in an attempt to control their own destinies. It should come as little surprise, then, to see that independence, autonomy, egalitarianism and self-determinism are celebrated ideals that point to a common world view and value pattern shared between mainstream rehabilitation ideology and the broader Western social contexts that raised them (Iwama 2004).

One distinct feature commonly seen in East Asian and Aboriginal world views is that the 'self' is not central nor unilaterally empowered but rather construed to be just one of many parts of an inseparable whole (Bellah 1991, Gustafson 1993). In this view of reality, one does not need to occupy nor wrest control of anything because, in an integrated view of self and nature, one is already there among others. Health and disability states are also not imagined nor believed to be an individual-centred matter. Life circumstances are dependent on a broader whole, determined by a constellation of factors and elements located both within and outside the physically defined body. The self is decentralised and not accorded exclusive privilege to exercise stewardship or unilateral control over one's environment or circumstances. Hence, conceptual models of rehabilitation that are based on a tacit understanding of a central individual separate from a discrete environment may not adequately explain experiences of disability, health and rehabilitation for many who are situated outside mainstream Western social norms.

Self in relation to time: implications for rehabilitation

Where and how *self* is imagined to be situated in relation to the environment also has a bearing on how views of life and the world are temporally constructed. In Eastern philosophies and in many Aboriginal narratives, where self is often not experienced as situated in a central, privileged position of reference, one's temporal orientation tends to coincide with the sensation of being situated in the present, or here-and-now. A state of wellness is reached when all elements in a frame, including the self, co-exist in harmony. Disruption of this harmony hampers the collective synergy or life-flow/energy. 'Enhancing or restoring harmony' supplants self-determinism and unilateral control as the primary purpose for occupational therapy and rehabilitation in many non-Western contexts. This partially explains why rehabilitation care recipients and therapists situated outside Western social experience find the core meanings and philosophical reasons behind their rehabilitation treatments difficult at times to understand and to reconcile to their own realities. The theory and philosophy is perplexing and does not resonate with their own cultural values and imperatives around wellbeing. In the worst cases, rehabilitative therapies as they are understood in the Western world can appear incongruous and asynchronous with local people's ideas of wellbeing and health. Not surprisingly then, in these non-Western settings, rehabilitative approaches such as occupational therapy have been reduced to a more mechanical and medical definition, and are largely understood and delivered in pathology- or medical illness-focused, recipe-style, interventions within the contexts of the culture and practices of Western biomedicine.

Owing to the cultural context-bound nature of existing rehabilitation theory, conceptual models founded on alternative cultural world views are crucially required but unfortunately have been largely absent until now.

THE KAWA MODEL

Origins

The *Kawa* Model was raised from an Asian occupational therapy practice context through a process of qualitative research that took place in the late 1990s. Frustrated and discouraged by trying to understand and apply imported occupational therapy and rehabilitation theory into their own practices, a group of Japanese occupational therapists decided to develop their own conceptual model of practice with the help of a Japanese–Canadian occupational therapist–social scientist.

Particularly troubling to these rehabilitation clinicians in Japan were the rugged-individual-oriented values and social imperatives imbedded in imported theories, which were difficult to adapt to their own familiar form of social collectivism. The imported Western ideas were intriguing at first but all too frequently conflicted with their own value patterns and social norms around matters of health and wellness in day-to-day experience. The future-oriented, rational explanations of individual agency, seen in the rehabilitation goals for client autonomy and independence, were practically impossible for – even offensive to – the local clientele, which for generations had adhered to a more integrated, naturalistic, socially interdependent view of reality. Having no existing models that were culturally relevant to Eastern world views to adapt or use as a base for an alternative approach, these Japanese occupational therapists proceeded to explore alternative ways to reconcile theory with their practice realities.

They first attempted to make better translations of the original concepts of existing occupational therapy models ,but ultimately this was not enough as they began to understand that there were substantial differences in the social and cultural contexts supporting the meanings of the concepts and principles contained in these models. If the (Western) meanings and merits of autonomy, self determinism, rugged American individualism, etc., could not be adequately grasped and imagined from the (Eastern) experience and vantage of hierarchically structured collectivism, the validity and utility of these theories and the very idea of occupational therapy itself were threatened.

Without theoretical material that made sense to the average Japanese person's world of everyday experience and meaning, Japanese occupational therapy was on the brink of a professional crisis. An absence of understandable and culturally meaningful occupational therapy theory over the span of three decades had resulted in a practice that had become increasingly reliant on biomechanical and medical-pathology-centred models. Japanese occupational therapists felt discouraged and disillusioned by what amounted to a profession defined by impairment-centred techniques and assessments. Professional identity and morale were lagging as occupational therapists had difficulty articulating their roles on their interdisciplinary rehabilitation teams.

The group set about examining the basis of their practice and began to work toward developing an alternative model of occupational therapy to better inform their rehabilitation practice. In the process, they were led through an exercise of discussing their culturally situated views of what was essential to their lives, including their sense of wellness and their definitions and understanding of illness, health and disability. They were challenged to articulate what they and their clients lived for, what was essential to life and fulfilment, in order to redefine occupation and realign the purpose of occupational therapy to matters of essential importance to the Japanese person's life and world.

The research initially led to a cumbersome representation of their model along conventional, linear box and arrow structures (Fig. 8.1). At that early stage, it became readily apparent that there were fundamental differences in how self and environment were imagined and *lived*. For a model to purposely explain self and context, the central placement of a distinctly defined self adjacent to a separate but distinct environment, commonly seen in conventional (Western) models, was non-existent. Further consideration revealed comprehension of self and environment or context that was more diffuse and inseparably integrated by the Japanese than by their Western counterparts.

Consistent with a world view that imagined self and the world and all of its elements as integrated parts of an all-encompassing whole, phenomena as complex as wellbeing and disability could not be adequately described and explained by linear diagrams that connected rationally defined categories through logical principles. This Eastern perspective of wellness and disability states could not be readily contained in and explained by boxes/categories set in a logical sequence in a rational formula or continuum.

In this initial diagram, what was effectively captured was the interconnectedness of all elements and phenomena in the frame of life experience; that states of wellbeing and disability are neither internally (in the body) nor externally (in the environment) isolated. The self and environment were inextricably connected in a manner in which a change in one component would effect a change in the greater whole. Observers who wonder why there is a Japanese social tendency to conform to group norms, or to not be the metaphorical nail that stands up (needing to be hammered down) are encouraged to consider this particular world view, in which balance and harmony are founded on the integration of all parts of a dynamic whole.

Figure 8.1 Initial attempt at a Japanese model of occupational therapy.

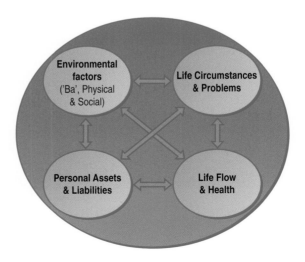

Although this framework effectively represented the East Asian conceptualisation of a diffuse self, unified, interdependent with and inseparable from other elements in the environment, the form of this representation still was not considered an adequate portrayal of Eastern views of life. During a subsequent session, the research participants decided to employ a metaphor of nature (a river, or *kawa* in Japanese) to better explain the dynamic and fluid nature of the model. The use of such a metaphor contrasted dramatically with the familiar mechanical and 'system' metaphors frequently employed in the construction of Western conceptual models.

Structure and components of the Kawa Model

The complex dynamic that characterises an Eastern perspective of harmony in life experience between self and context might be best explained through a familiar metaphor (Lakoff et al 1980) of nature. Life is a complex, profound journey that flows through time and space, like a river (Fig. 8.2). An optimal state of wellbeing in one's life, or river, can be metaphorically portrayed by an image of strong, deep, unimpeded flow. Aspects of the environment and phenomenal circumstances, like certain structures found in a river, can influence and affect that flow. Rocks (life circumstances), walls and bottom (environment), driftwood (assets and liabilities) are all inseparable parts of a river that determine its boundaries, shape, flow rate and overall quality (Fig. 8.3). Occupational therapy's purpose, then, in concert with an interdisciplinary rehabilitation mandate, is to enable and enhance life flow by enhancing harmony (between all elements that form the overall context).

Figure 8.2 Life is like a river, flowing from birth to end of life.

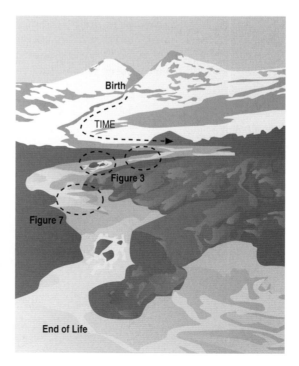

Figure 8.3 At any given point along its continuum, a cross-section of the river can be considered, to understand life's condition from the client's vantage point. The quality of water flow is affected by the river walls and bottom, rocks and driftwood. Whenever there is a need to enhance life flow, there is a need for occupational therapy.

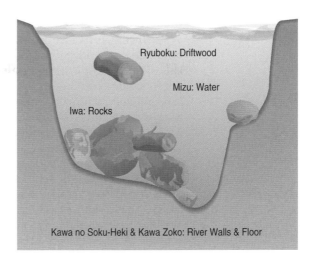

Ryuboku: Driftwood

Mizu: Water

Iwa: Rocks

Kawa no Soku-Heki & Kawa Zoko: River Walls & Floor

Water (mizu)

Mizu – Japanese for 'water', metaphorically represents the subject's life energy or life flow. Fluid, pure, spirit, filling, cleansing and renewing, are only some of the meanings and functions commonly associated with this natural element. Just as people's lives are bounded and shaped by their surroundings, people and circumstances, the water flowing as a river touches the rocks, sides and banks and all other elements that form its context. Water envelopes, defines and affects these other elements of the river in a similar way to which the same elements affect the water's volume, shape and flow rate.

When life energy or the water flow weakens, the client – whether individually or collectively defined – can be described as unwell, or in a state of disharmony. When it stops flowing altogether, as when the river releases into a vast ocean, end of life is reached.

Just as water is fluid and adopts its form from its container, people in many collectively oriented societies often interpret the social as a shaper of individual self. Sharing a view of the cosmos that embeds the self inextricably within the environment, collectively oriented people tend to place enormous value on the self embedded in relationships. There is greater value in 'belonging' and 'interdependence' than in unilateral agency and in individual determinism (Nakane 1970, Doi 1973, Lebra 1976). In such experience, the interdependent self is deeply influenced and even determined by the surrounding social context, at a given time and place, in a similar way to that in which water in a river, at any given point, varies in form, flow direction, rate volume and clarity. The 'driving force' of one's life is interconnected with others sharing the same social frame or *ba* (Nakane 1970), in a similar way in which water is seen to touch, connect and relate all elements of a river that have varying effect upon its form and flow.

With so much focused on the independent and agent self, there may be a tendency to overlook or underestimate the importance that place and context plays in determining the form, functions and meanings of human occupation. From the vantage of the *Kawa* Model, a subject's state of wellbeing coincides with life-flow. Occupational therapy's and rehabilitation's overall purpose in this context is to enhance life flow, regardless of whether it is interpreted at the level of the individual, institution, organisation, community or society. Just as there are constellations of inter-related factors/structures in a river that affect its flow, a rich combination of internal and external circumstances and structures in a client's life context inextricably determine his or her life flow.

River side–walls and river bottom (kawa no soku–heki and kawa no zoko)

The river's sides and bottom, referred to in the Japanese lexicon respectively as *kawa no soku-heki* and *kawa no zoko*, are the structures/concepts from the river metaphor that represent the client's environment. These are perhaps the most important determinants of a person's life flow in a collectivist social context because of the primacy accorded to the environmental context in determining the construction of self, experience of being and subsequent meanings of personal action. In the *Kawa* Model, the river walls and sides represent the subject's social context – mainly those people who share a direct relationship with the subject. Depending upon which social frame is perceived as being most important in a given instance and place, the river sides and bottom can represent family members, workmates, friends in a recreational club, classmates, etc. In certain non-Western societies, such as that of Japan, social relationships are regarded to be the central determinant (Nakane1970) of individual and collective life flow.

Aspects of the surrounding social frame on the subject can affect the overall flow (volume and rate) of the *kawa*. Harmonious relationships can enable and complement life flow. Increased flow can have an agent effect upon difficult circumstances and problems as the force of water displaces rocks in the channel and even creates new courses through which to flow. Conversely, a decrease in flow volume can exert a compounding, negative effect on the other elements that take up space in the channel (Fig. 8.4). If there are obstructions (rocks and driftwood) in the watercourse when the river walls and bottom are thick and constricting, the flow of the river is especially compromised. As can readily be imagined, the rocks in this river can directly butt up against the river walls and bottom, compounding and creating larger impediments to the river's usual flow. When applying the *Kawa* Model in collectivist-oriented populations, these components and the perceptions of their importance are paramount.

Like all other elements of the river, these concepts are always interpreted in relation to the whole, taking into consideration all other elements of the subject's context and their interrelations/interdependencies.

Rocks (iwa)

Iwa (Japanese for large rocks or crags) represent discrete circumstances that are considered to be impediments to one's life flow. They are life circumstances perceived by the client to be problematic and difficult to remove. Every rock, like every life circumstance, has a unique size, density, shape, colour and texture. Most rivers, like people's lives, have such rocks or impediments, of varying quality and number. Large rocks, by

Figure 8.4 The shape and status of the water, or life flow, is determined by the compounding interplay of rocks (problems), driftwood (assets/liabilities) and the river walls and floor (environment). Rocks increase in size, shape and number, situated along a dynamic, enclosing environment, trapping driftwood, Life flow is compromised, indicating a need for occupational therapy.

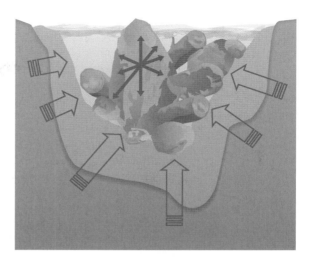

themselves or in combination with other rocks, jammed directly or indirectly against the river walls and sides (environment) can profoundly impede and obstruct flow. The client's rocks may have been there since the beginning, as with congenital conditions. They may appear instantaneously, as in sudden illness or injury, and even be transient.

The impeding effect of rocks can be compounded when they are situated against the river's sides and walls (environment). A person's bodily impairment becomes disabling when interfaced with the environment. For example, the functional difficulties associated with a neurological condition can change according to the environmental context. A (physically) barrier-free environment can decrease one's disability, as can a social and/or political/organisational environment that is accepting of people with disabling conditions. Once the client's perceived rocks are known (including their relative size and situation), the therapist can help to identify potential areas of intervention and strategies to enable better life flow. The broader contextual definition of disabling circumstances necessarily brings into play the client's surrounding environment. Although often limited to narrow, medically oriented interventions in hospital institutions, occupational therapy intervention can therefore include treatment strategies that expand beyond the traditional patient to his or her social network and even to policies and social structures of the surrounding institution or society that ultimately play a part in setting the disabling context.

The concepts and the contextual application of the *Kawa* Model are, by natural design, flexible and adaptable. Each client's unique river takes its important concepts and configuration from the situation of the subject, in a given time and place. The definitions of problems and circumstances are broad – as broad and diverse as the rehabilitation clients' worlds of meanings. In turn, this particular conceptualisation of people and their circumstances foreshadows the broad outlook and scope of occupational therapy interventions when set in particular cultural contexts.

The subject, be it an individual or a collective, ideally determines specific rocks, their number, magnitude, quality and situation in the river. As with all other elements of the model, if the client is unable to express their own river, family members or a community of people connected with the issues may lend assistance and perspective.

Driftwood (ryuboku)

Ryuboku is Japanese for 'driftwood' and, in the context of the *Kawa* Model, represents the subject's personal attributes and resources, such as values (e.g. honesty, thrift), character (e.g. optimism, stubbornness), personality (e.g. reserved, outgoing), special skill (e.g. carpentry, public speaking), immaterial assets (e.g. friends, siblings) and material assets (e.g. wealth, special equipment), which can positively or negatively affect the subject's circumstance and life flow.

Like driftwood, they are transient in nature and carry a certain quality of fate or serendipity. They can appear to be inconsequential in some instances and significantly obstructive in others – particularly when they settle in among rocks and the river-sides and walls. On the other hand, they can collide with the same structures to nudge obstructions out of the way. A client's religious faith and sense of determination can be positive factors in persevering to erode or move rocks out of the way. For example, receiving a monetary gift or donation to acquire specialised assistive equipment can be the piece of driftwood that collides against existing flow impediments and opens a greater channel for one's life to flow more strongly.

Driftwood is a part of everyone's river and often includes those intangible components possessed by each unique rehabilitation client. Effective therapists pay particular attention to these components of a client's or community's assets and circumstances and consider their real or potential effect on the client's situation.

Space between obstructions (sukima); the promise of occupational therapy

In the *Kawa* Model, spaces are the points through which the client's life energy (water) evidently flows, and these spaces represent 'occupation', in an East Asian perspective. When the metaphor of a river depicting the client's life flow becomes clearer, attention turns to the *sukima* (spaces between the rocks, driftwood, and river walls and bottom). These spaces are as important to comprehend in the client's context as are the other elements of the river when determining how to apply and direct occupational therapy and rehabilitation. For example, a space between a functional impairment such as arthritis (an *iwa*/rock) and a social group or person (in the river sides and walls) may represent a certain social role, such as parent, company worker, friend, etc.

Water naturally coursing through these spaces can work to erode the rocks and river walls and bottom and over time transform them into larger conduits for life flow (Fig. 8.5). This effect reflects the latent healing potential that each subject naturally holds within their self and in the inseparable context. Thus occupational therapy in this perspective retains its hallmark of purposeful activity and working with the client's abilities and assets. It also directs occupational therapy intervention toward all elements (in this case; a medically defined problem,

Figure 8.5 *Sukima*/spaces: potential focal points for occupational therapy. Intervention can be multifaceted and include breaking or eroding away the (medical) problem, limiting personal liabilities and/or maximising personal assets, as well as intervening on elements of the greater environment (including the social and physical). Focusing water on these objects to erode or move them is metaphorical of the client using their own abilities or 'life force'.

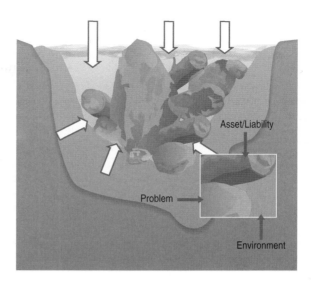

various aspects and levels of environment) in the context (see inner image, Fig. 8.5).

Spaces, then, represent important foci for occupational therapy and the broader rehabilitation effort. They occur throughout the context of the self and environs; between the rocks, walls and bottom, and driftwood. Spaces subsume the environment as part of the greater context of the problem and expands the scope of intervention to naturally integrate what, in the Western sense, would have been treated separately through the dualism of internal (pertaining to self and personal attributes) and external (environment constructed as separate and outside of the self). Spaces are potential channels for the client's flow, allowing client and therapist to determine multiple points and levels of intervention (Fig. 8.5). In this way, each problem or enabling opportunity is bounded by and appreciated in a broader context.

Rather than attempting to reduce a person's problems to discrete issues, isolated out of their particular contexts (i.e. focusing only on rocks), similar to the rational processes in which client problems are identified and discretely named/diagnosed in conventional Western health practice, the *Kawa* Model framework compels the occupational therapist and rehabilitation professional to view and treat issues within a holistic framework, seeking to appreciate the clients' identified issues within their integrated, inseparable contexts. Occupation is therefore regarded in wholes – to include the meaning of the activity to self and community to which the individual inseparably belongs, and not just in terms of biomechanical components, or individual pathology and function.

Phenomena and life circumstances rarely occur in isolation. By changing one aspect of the client's world, all other aspects of their river change. The river's spaces represent opportunities to problem-solve and focus intervention on positive opportunities, which may have little direct relation to the person's medically defined condition.

By using this model, occupational therapists, in partnership with their clients, are directed to stem further obstruction of life energy/flow and look for every opportunity in the broader context to enhance it (Figs 8.6, 8.7).

Harmony: the essence of human occupation and a reconceptualisation of rehabilitation

What has been described is the underlying ontology of the *Kawa* framework. The kawa model's central point of reference is not the individual but rather harmony – a state of individual or collective being in which the subject, be it self or community, is in balance with the context that it is a part of. Here, the essence of such harmony is conceptualised as 'life energy' or 'life flow'. Occupational therapy's purpose, in concert with the mandate of rehabilitation, is to help the client and community

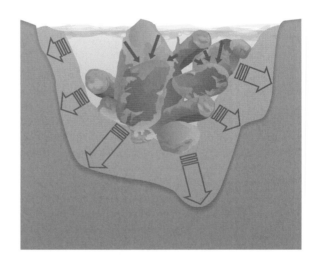

Figure 8.6 Occupational therapy helps to identify spaces where water (life force) can still flow and focuses water through the spaces, over rocks (problems/obstacles), driftwood (resources; liabilities and assets) and floor/sides (environmental context), eroding the surfaces and thus increasing life flow.

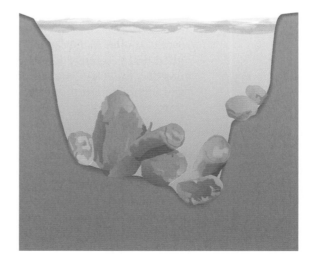

Figure 8.7 The power of occupational therapy: increased life flow. All obstacles may not have been completely eliminated; some may even have remained unchanged. however, *life* flows more strongly, despite life's obstacles and challenges.

enhance and balance this flow. In this balance, there is co-existence, a synergy between elements that affirm interdependence. How can one come to terms with one's circumstances? How can harmony between the elements, of which one is merely a part, be realised? How and in what way can occupational therapists and their interdisciplinary partners assist this construction of wellbeing?

EMPLOYMENT OF THE KAWA METAPHOR IN REHABILITATION PRACTICE

The *Kawa* Model represents a novel addition to conventional occupational therapy conceptual model development in a number of ways. To begin with, the *Kawa* Model is explicitly described as a culturally situated product, having been raised out of an Asian social context. The model is also peculiar in regard to its structure, diverging from conventional scientific, rational form, taking the shape of a common metaphor of nature.

For many, the river is a familiar metaphor for 'life'. This construct of life as a fluid continuum situated in nature is congruent with certain Eastern philosophical and ethical systems such as Buddhism (particularly Mahayana and Zen), Confucianism and Taoism. Similarities and congruities as well as differences in interpretations of the river metaphor are bound to exist and will therefore be applicable in one form or another for some and inappropriate for others. Like people's experiences of wellness and disability, there is no one standard explanation or norm. In cases where the model cannot be adequately adapted to suit the client's construction of his or her state of wellbeing, or when the river metaphor holds less explanatory power in the client's context, the model should be placed aside for a more fitting alternative. Therefore, all universal assumptions and proprietary interpretations of the model and its applicability are dismissed, permitting and encouraging occupational therapists to alter and adapt the model in conceptual and structural ways to match the specific social and cultural contexts of their diverse clients.

Although the *Kawa* Model may appear to favour Japanese cultural contexts, it should not be viewed as culturally exclusive. The utility and safety of this model for varying populations depends on the river metaphor's familiarity and relevance to its subjects. The *Kawa* Model has been introduced to groups of practitioners in a variety of cultural settings spanning three continents (Okuda et al 2000, Hibino et al 2002, Iwama et al 2002, Fujimoto et al 2003, Iwama & Fujimoto 2003), with encouraging results. Occupational therapists should view the *Kawa* Model as a tool to better understand and appreciate their clients' complex occupational circumstances.

While the benefits of the *Kawa* Model as an effective tool within occupational therapy are being explored, there is already some evidence pointing to its interprofessional utility. The power of the river metaphor is familiar not only to many rehabilitation clients but also to members of the interdisciplinary rehabilitation care team. As each team member carries his or her own unique professional perspective of the client's issues and expertise in helping to ameliorate identified problems, assistance is sometimes needed to connect each professional vantage and intervention to the client's whole context. Given the highly specialised and complex meanings of concepts in the language of each health-care profession, a common metaphor that is understandable across health disciplines (and to the client) is potentially useful. How does a physiotherapist understand how their complex cranial–sacral treatment intervention integrates with what the occupational therapist calls occupational performance, and how does it all fit into the overall context of the client's return to participation in normal life situations?

Employing a simple metaphor like the *Kawa* to communicate how each professional's intervention fits into the client's life situation and rehabilitation plan can be very useful. The *Kawa* Model can potentially tie each rehabilitation professional's mandate into the larger context of the client's care plan in a client-centred way. Nishihama et al (2002) found, in their prospective study of three cases where the *Kawa* Model was used to discuss and coordinate rehabilitation client issues across health disciplines, that the river metaphor demonstrated promise as both a communication and a coordinating tool. Nishihama et al found that not only did non-occupational-therapists appreciate (some reportedly for the very first time) occupational therapy's scope of practice and mandate in these cases, but that the clarification of each profession's role in enhancing the client's 'life flow' resulted in better coordination and service delivery to the client. Although further studies are warranted to determine whether the use of the *Kawa* Model results in better rehabilitation outcomes, the potential use of such models to serve as a common language in explicating the complexities of comprehensive rehabilitation care to both client and the rehabilitation team should not be overlooked.

A client–centred perspective and practice

To be truly client-centred, the client's views of their realities and circumstances should not be forced to comply with someone else's manufactured framework of rigid concepts and principles. The therapist using the *Kawa* Model recognises, first, the uniqueness of each subject's situation/context. The structure and meanings of the river metaphor take shape according to the subject's views of their circumstances in a particular cultural context. Rehabilitation professionals may overlook the cultural limitations of conventional client-centred approaches. They should be aware that client-centred approaches are often shaped and delivered through an individualist ideology that tacitly advances the ideals of individual autonomy and self efficacy that is considered normal in Western cultural experience.

Therefore, one uses the *Kawa* metaphor to derive concepts that are meaningful and germane to the client's perspective of life and wellbeing. As the client's unique concepts and issues are determined, the therapist goes about selecting tools/instruments and methods that will effectively gather pertinent information. These chosen instruments should also be culturally safe and non-exploitative. Equipped with the *Kawa* framework, the occupational therapist does not become dependent on a particular measurement tool or procedure to inform them what their

CASE STUDY SHELLY

Shelly is 27 and works for a law firm in the city. She graduated with a first class honours degree from her university and is considered a 'high flyer' in her field. Her family are living in Canada and she travels to see them frequently. She has a wide circle of friends and for the past year has been seeing Jonathan, who works for the same firm. It was while she was on a winter sports holiday in Europe with Jonathan that she had a skiing accident, which left her with spinal cord injuries. As a result of this she has a spinal cord lesion at T10. After spending some time in a European hospital while her condition was stabilised, she has now flown back to a spinal injuries unit, where she has been receiving rehabilitation. The team working with Shelly have noticed her becoming more and more withdrawn since her admission, and she has been talking to them about how hopeless she feels and that she wishes her life would end.

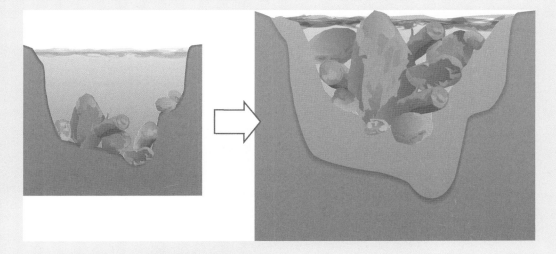

Using the river metaphor as a framework to understand more profoundly the contextual nature of Shelly's difficulties and challenges from her perspective, we begin to appreciate the multifaceted and complex dimensions of her experience of life in the present, which will have a profound bearing on her rehabilitation.

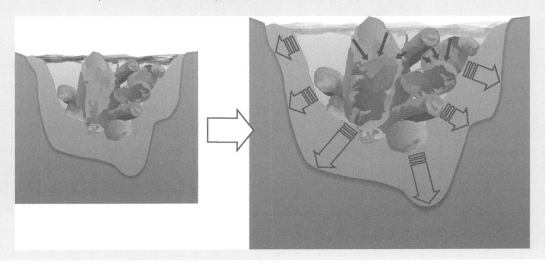

For example, we find that Shelly is consumed by the full impact of her condition on her life and future. The vibrant and hopeful life she led has been betrayed by this sudden, unforeseeable spinal cord injury and its overwhelming consequences. While the health team are hard at work stabilising her injury, determining the extent of her impairment and exploring ways to restore as much functional performance as possible, Shelly sees her life as she knew and wanted it completely erased, leaving her with a sense of fear, diminished self-esteem and worth, and pessimism about her future life.

Her life energy (water) has been robbed from her; her river increasingly impeded by a host of interrelated, compounding barriers. Privately, she thinks to herself: 'Will I ever walk again? Who will employ a person in my condition? Good-bye Jonathan, good-bye to marriage, to children, the lot. How will I live? Will my friends . . . who will want me for a friend? How will I manage from day to day? I'm finished.'

Shelly's river (life-force) is flowing weakly. The impedance to flow is due to a complex connection of numerous factors (physical, social, political, medical) that are interconnected.

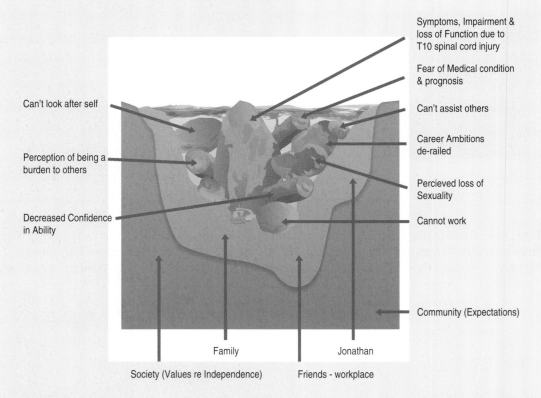

Symptoms, Impairment & loss of Function due to T10 spinal cord injury

Fear of Medical condition & prognosis

Can't look after self

Can't assist others

Career Ambitions de-railed

Perception of being a burden to others

Percieved loss of Sexuality

Decreased Confidence in Ability

Cannot work

Community (Expectations)

Family   Jonathan

Society (Values re Independence)   Friends - workplace

Using the river framework to explicate the complex context of Shelly's circumstances, the occupational therapist, together with the team, begins to identify those channels where Shelly's life (water) continues to flow. These channels are bounded by her perceived problems and challenges (rocks) residual abilities and liabilities (driftwood) and aspects of her physical and social environment (river floor and sides). Intervention, like Shelly's circumstances, is multifaceted, involving a combination of foci and approaches and the full participation of the interdisciplinary team. Rocks, in the immediate time frame, might be eroded through activities of daily living training and education about her condition. The social. psychological and spiritual consequences of her spinal cord injury emerge fully from Shelly's river narrative and deserve primary attention. Profound issues of sexuality and future potential/loss might be approached through psychological counselling and social work interventions. Walls and bottom might be expanded by family and client discussions to facilitate greater understanding and support for Shelly. Counselling involving Shelly and Jonathan may be an option.

Special equipment and modifications to Shelly's home environment might be targeted to enable greater ability. As the river contents and structure expand, the channels become wider and Shelly's life-force is liberated to flow more strongly and fully. The essence of occupational therapy is to enhance life flow. In this way, occupational therapy is comprehensive, integrated with other rehabilitation services, contextual and client-centred. As more information emerges about the characteristics of Shelly's river, the intervention becomes more profound and focused.

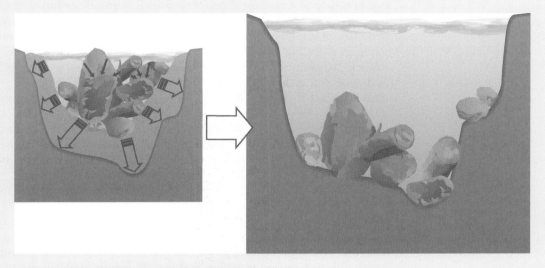

This is merely a simplified case vignette to demonstrate the use of the river metaphor. Practitioners around the world are beginning to find that the model is useful in applications beyond the individual: to collectives, communities and organisations.

interventions ought to be. Rather, the therapist is challenged and guided toward understanding the clients' occupational and rehabilitative issues in their proper context to gain a clearer sense of what needs to be measured and studied further, and why. The instruments and tools are chosen judiciously according to the requirements of the client's case, in proper context, set in harmony with the overall rehabilitation mandate.

DISCUSSION

Clients participating in rehabilitation treatment are rarely socially and culturally homogeneous. Each client brings a unique configuration of personal attributes coupled with a unique set of contextual conditions.

Consequently, the formula for wellness and the structure and experience of disability are just as unique and specific to each client's case. What is considered to be disabling in one context may be less or more so in another. Universally applicable theoretical precepts that carry social imperatives, such as autonomy and independence, or classification systems that reduce the complexities of human experience to rational categories, have their own advantages and disadvantages. On the one hand, they may help rehabilitation professionals to standardise matters of wellness and disability and help to ensure a better level of care across a broad international spectrum. However, on the other hand, these classifications may also lead to disadvantaging those who fall toward the margins or even outside of a classification framework's normal categories. As rehabilitation practice continues its foray into new cultural frontiers, the diversity of contexts in which people define what is important and of value in daily life in relation to their states of wellbeing will only continue to broaden. Beyond race and ethnicity, conditions of poverty, limited access to technology, a global economy, diversity in health policy, continuation of population migration and deprivation of meaningful participation in society, to name but a few, represent some real-world contexts for the lives of millions of people. These increasingly familiar contexts will challenge the meaning and efficacy of occupational therapy and the meaning of rehabilitation in this era. Can the ICF adequately meet these diverse social and cultural conditions?

Culture in the broader sense in which it has been presented in this chapter may very well be the next hurdle for the ICF to work its way through. Already, we are seeing the need for alterations to the framework to accommodate the varying 'cultural' conditions experienced by children (Simeonsson et al 2003). Will advocates for people representing various collective experiences in matters of health and disability also petition for a more useful and equitable variant of the universal classification framework? Time will tell. In the meantime, models like the *Kawa* are offered to help comprehend the particular and culturally specific features of people's disability experiences – particularly for those clients whose life contexts fall outside the explanatory powers of models emerged from mainstream Western social contexts.

The Japanese occupational therapists who raised the *Kawa* Model from their day-to-day practice seek to remind their international colleagues of the primacy and importance of nature as context, and how its laws need to be more fundamentally apparent in our epistemology, theory and practice in rehabilitation. The rhythms and cycles of nature continue to prevail and have yet to yield to mankind's attempts to transcend and subjugate them. In the Eastern perspective of humanity integrated in nature, occupational therapy may be appreciated less as an empowerment or enablement of the individual's dominion over nature and circumstance, but as an empowerment of bringing individuals' life forces into harmony and better flow with nature and its circumstances. As long as there is a need for harmony between self and context, there is then a need for culturally relevant rehabilitation and occupational therapy.

Along with the acknowledgement of the primacy of nature in human experience, the *Kawa* Model also serves as a prototype for a new way of regarding and employing theoretical material in our rehabilitation professions. In this postmodern era of recognising cultural relativity, variation in world-views and interpretations of life, the notion of one rigid explanation of function and wellbeing will be increasingly difficult to retain. The same difficulty applies to occupational therapists and the meanings of their concept of occupation in a broader sense as it relates to meaningful activity in daily life. The notion of a universal explanation for occupation would potentially limit occupational therapy's cultural relevance and meaning to a narrower exclusive scope of practice. The same might also apply to other rehabilitation professional groups and their respective interests.

Occupational therapy and rehabilitation, in an ideal sense, should be as unique as its clients – changing its form and approach according to the clients' diverse circumstances and meanings of wellbeing. To move closer to that ideal, conceptual models and theory in rehabilitation should be better informed and drawn, at least in part, from diverse social landscapes and profound contents of the therapist-client practice context.

QUESTIONS FOR DISCUSSION

- In what ways is culture expressed in your professional practice?
- What are some of the cultural features imbedded in the structure and content in familiar rehabilitation theory and models?
- To what extent is culture taken into account in client-centred approaches in rehabilitation?
- Using the river metaphor outlined in this chapter, construct your own river diagram to depict your current state of being. How might you adapt elements of your river to enhance your 'life flow'?

References

Bellah R 1991 Beyond belief: essays on religion in a post traditional world. Harper & Row, New York

Canadian Association of Occupational Therapists 2003 Enabling occupation: an occupational therapy perspective, 2nd edn. CAOT Publications, Toronto

Doi T 1973 The anatomy of dependence. Kodansha International, Tokyo

Fujimoto H., Yoshimura N, Iwama M 2003 The *Kawa* (River) Model workshop – addressing diversity of culture in occupational therapy. 3rd Asia Pacific Occupational Therapy Congress, Singapore

Gustafson JM 1993 Man and nature: a cross-cultural perspective. Chulalongkorn University Press, Bangkok

Hibino K, Tanaka M, Iwama M et al 2002 Applying a new model of Japanese occupational therapy to a client case of depression. 13th International Congress of the World Federation of Occupational Therapists, Stockholm

Iwama M 2003 The issue is . . . toward culturally relevant epistemologies in occupational therapy. American Journal of Occupational Therapy 57:582–588

Iwama M 2004 Situated meaning: an issue of culture, inclusion and occupational therapy. In: Kronenberg F, Algado SA., Pollard N (eds) Occupational therapy without borders – learning from the spirit of survivors. Churchill Livingstone, Edinburgh

Iwama M Fujimoto H 2003 How does your river flow? Using a culturally relevant model of occupational therapy to break through occupational barriers. Occupational Therapy Atlantic Conference 2003, Oak Island, Canada

Iwama M, Hatsutori T, Okuda M 2002 Emerging a culturally and clinically relevant conceptual model of Japanese occupational therapy. 13th International Congress of the World Federation of Occupational Therapists, Stockholm

Kielhofner GA 2002 Model of human occupation: theory and application, 3rd edn. Williams & Wilkins, Baltimore

Lakoff G, Johnson M 1980 Metaphors we live by. University of Chicago Press, Chicago

Lebra S 1976 Japanese patterns of behavior. University of Hawaii Press, Honolulu

Nakane C 1970 Tate shakai no ningen kankei [Human relations in a vertical society]. Kodansha, Tokyo

Nishihama M, Koushima H, Iwama M 2002 Explaining occupational therapy to health teams; benefits of a culturally relevant model. Poster. 13th International Congress of the World Federation of Occupational Therapists, Stockholm

Okuda M, Iwama M, Hatsutori T et al 2000 A Japanese model of occupational therapy; One; the 'river model' raised from the clinical setting. Journal of the Japanese Association of Occupational Therapists 19(suppl):512

Simeonsson RJ, Leonardi M, Bjorck-Akesson E et al 2003 Measurement of disability in children and youth: implications of the ICF. Disability and Rehabilitation 25:602–610

Smith MJ 2000 Culture: reinventing the social sciences. Open University Press, Buckingham

World Health Organization 2001 International Classification of Functioning, Disability and Health. WHO, Geneva

Chapter **9**

The Way Forward

Sally Davis

INTRODUCTION

The aim of this book has been to consider the use of different types of model in rehabilitation and to identify how they can promote interprofessional working. Perhaps one of the key developments over the last 2 years that is significant to rehabilitation is the revision of the International Classification of Impairments, Disability and Handicaps (World Health Organization 1980). This has resulted in the ICF: International Classification of Functioning, Disability and Health (World Health Organization 2002). There is a need for further development of the ICF and further consideration as to how it can be used in practice. Hopefully this book will have taken the discussion forward as to how the ICF can be used in rehabilitation and how it links in with other models looking at concepts related to rehabilitation. The aim of this chapter is to:

- Summarise the main points of the book
- Identify areas for future development and research
- Identify implications for interprofessional training.

REHABILITATION

One of the issues about rehabilitation is that it is extremely complex, with a number of concepts impacting on it such as multi- or interdisciplinary team working, adaptation, health promotion, goal planning, client-centredness, quality of life, advocacy, empowerment, enablement, independence, occupation. Using one model to guide practice will not pick up on this complexity. The ICF has value in that it provides rehabilitation professionals with a structure to consider aspects of the individual in context, for example body systems, body functions, functional outcomes, personal factors, environmental factors (Spencer et al 2002). However, it is limited in that it doesn't take into account the total experience for the individual (Wade & Halligan 2003). Maybe one of the issues is that the ICF is a classification rather than a conceptual model. Therefore using the ICF in conjunction with other models can assist rehabilitation professionals to really be holistic practitioners. In my experience there are areas related to individuals' quality of life that rehabilitation professionals do not address well, for example sexual wellbeing, spirituality, culture and health promotion. Using a combination of models can give rehabilitation professionals tools and guidance on how to assess and manage all aspects that will affect an individual's quality of life.

Uniprofessional models are used consistently among the professions; however, there is little evidence of these models being considered in an interprofessional way. The way forward perhaps is for us to really consider how models can be used to promote interprofessional working and used to really address the issues for individuals as they go through the rehabilitation process. If rehabilitation is to be meaningful for the individual then it is important that professionals are able to recognise what this means and to consider the concepts that may affect this process. The ICF goes some way in helping professionals consider not only physical functioning but also contextual factors in terms of the environment and attitudes. There is also recognition of personal factors, although it is not clear what these are. Using other models in conjunction with the ICF can perhaps highlight what these may be, for example:

- *The Canadian Model* (Ch. 4) considers the impact of occupation on the individual and what personal factors affect it. It highlights the relationship between the person, environment and occupations they have and have had. It also identifies spirituality as being that which makes individuals unique
- *The Illness Constellation Model* (Ch. 5) considers where the individual is in terms of taking control and seeking closure and where their significant others are in the process. It helps identify what factors personal to the individual and their family may be impeding or assisting this process, for example locus of control, coping strategies, roles. It can also help focus on what motivates the individual and their significant others
- *The Ex-PLISSIT Model* (Ch. 6) helps identify personal issues for the individual related to their sexual wellbeing. It also considers the level of comfortableness for professionals in addressing sensitive issues
- *Health Promotion Models* (Ch. 7) focus on why individuals behave in certain ways, taking into account their values, sociocultural and religious beliefs. The concepts of empowerment and advocacy are key
- *The Kawa (River) Model* (Ch. 8) considers disability and health states in a particular dynamic way relating individuals to the cultural context in which they live. Appreciating the individual's experience from their perspective enables personal factors to be identified in the context of their impact for that individual.

One of the difficulties with models is that there is a view that they need to be followed prescriptively. If models are to assist professionals in their practice then they need to be appropriate to that practice, which may mean adapting them or using a combination of models. To consider which models are suited to different practice settings needs to start with the team considering what their philosophy of practice is. What are their beliefs around the individual (client), their significant others, the health-care professional, the environment, rehabilitation? How do these all interact with each other? It is these elements that most models are developed around. So it makes sense for the team to start from that point and then to consider which models fit their philosophy. Considering the question in this way can help the team consider from the outset how they can use the models to promote interprofessional working. This has been the rationale for this book in the models chosen. Not only have they been chosen to reflect different types of model but they have also been chosen because they reflect my beliefs about rehabilitation – that rehabilitation:

- Should be focused on quality of life for the individual
- Needs to be delivered using a multi- or interdisciplinary approach
- Must include individual-centred goal planning
- Needs to be focused on the individual's experience
- Needs to consider the context the individual is in, which includes the cultural and environmental context
- Should commence from the acute stage.

Focusing on these beliefs can help rehabilitation professionals move the focus away from illness and disability to health and wellness. This challenge needs to be embraced, and using a variety of models to consider different aspects related to health and wellness can assist rehabilitation professionals in doing this. The ICF perhaps is a move towards this, although, as the literature highlights (Wade & Halligan 2003), it needs more development and thought, particularly in how it addresses the concepts of quality of life, motivation and the influence of time on an individual's readiness to participate in the rehabilitation process.

This notion of models not being prescriptive leads on to the consideration of how they may be used in different ways. The PLISSIT model is a good example of this, being used almost exclusively to consider individuals' sexuality and sexual health-care needs. Yet it could be used just as well in the areas of loss and adaptation and spirituality, both areas that rehabilitation professionals may have difficulty in addressing. The extension of the PLISSIT model into the Ex-PLISSIT model is perhaps a good illustration of how existing models can be used and then developed by practitioners as a result of evaluation of their use. This identifies the importance of evaluating the models and adapting them accordingly. This may be in response to the changes in delivery of rehabilitation, for example, the move towards community rehabilitation and intermediate care in the UK.

FUTURE DEVELOPMENT AND RESEARCH

As already stated, there is a need for further development of the ICF, and already research into the different domains is being conducted (Heerkens et al 2003, Jette et al 2003, Parenboom & Chorus 2003, Ogonowski et al 2004). This research also needs to address the use of the

ICF with different diagnostic groups, for example, individuals with chronic illness, mental illness and acute illness. There is also a need for further research into interprofessional working in rehabilitation. Inter-disciplinary teamwork is identified in the literature as the way forward; however, there is little research to support its effectiveness. It would be good to see research into how models can promote interprofessional working. This would include the use of models seen as uniprofessional, for example, nursing, occupational therapy models. Perhaps the time has come to move away from promoting uniprofessional models to consid-ering their use for the whole team. Perhaps the focus should be on how they can assist the rehabilitation team in meeting the individual's goals and focus on their quality of life.

IMPLICATIONS FOR INTERPROFESSIONAL TRAINING

Uniprofessional models are considered in the education of health-care professionals but maybe the focus now needs to be on how models can promote interprofessional working. In educating rehabilitation profes-sionals, perhaps the place to start is to consider what rehabilitation is and the concepts it consists of. In my experience of developing and delivering a Baccalaureate and Masters programme in Rehabilitation (Box 9.1), I have learnt that rehabilitation professionals do not necessar-ily consider the theories underpinning it. The rehabilitation module I deliver as part of both programmes has been evaluated well by reha-bilitation professionals from different professional groups as enabling them to critically discuss rehabilitation concepts in relation to their own practice and to apply models and theories to their practice. The learning outcomes and content of the module could be seen as a framework for promoting interprofessional working in rehabilitation, with models as a key feature.

CONCLUSION

To enable rehabilitation to be truly focused on the individual, rehabilitation professionals need to understand the complexity of rehabilitation and know what tools are available to help them do this. There are already a number of models available that help explain different concepts related to rehabilita-tion and are developed to guide practice. Rehabilitation professionals need to be creative in how they apply these models and identify how they relate to their own philosophy of rehabilitation. The ICF is a useful tool for use in rehabilitation and examples are needed of how it is used in practice. There is also a need for further research into some of the concepts that underpin the rehabilitation process, for example interdisciplinary teamwork, quality of life, adaptation.

Box 9.1   Rehabilitation Module (S. Davis, School of Health and Social Care, Oxford Brookes University)

Learning outcomes

On completion of this module students will be able to:

- Critically discuss the implications of rehabilitation definitions, models and theoretical frameworks to practice
- Reflect on and critically discuss their own role in rehabilitation
- Reflect on and debate interprofessional working taking into account different types of team organisation and the roles of different disciplines
- Critically discuss the psycho-social effects of acute and chronic illness for the individual and their family and identify implications for the rehabilitation process taking into account cultural and diversity issues
- Critically discuss the evaluation of the effectiveness of rehabilitation
- Develop skills of critical appraisal and apply to rehabilitation research

Content

- *The individual's experience of the process*: Factors that affect role development, acute versus long-term rehabilitation, illness versus wellness, where does the individual stop being treated and start being rehabilitated, development and change of roles from acute care to rehabilitation
- *What is rehabilitation*: Definitions of rehabilitation: conducting a concept analysis to identify its attributes. Rehabilitation as a process and philosophy. The stages of rehabilitation
- *Models and theories*: Examining theoretical frameworks, e.g. systems theory, adaptation theory, motivational theory, and their relationship to rehabilitation. Critically discussing the ICF in relation to rehabilitation and its relationship to other models
- *Assessment in rehabilitation*: The role of assessment in rehabilitation. Critically discussing different assessment tools and their relevance to rehabilitation practice. Assessment in relation to the ICF and other models
- *The role of health promotion in rehabilitation*: Perceptions of health. Health promotion and the use of health promotion models. The relationship of empowerment to health promotion and rehabilitation
- *Working in a team*: Multidisciplinary, interdisciplinary and transdisciplinary approaches. Advantages and disadvantages of each approach in relation to rehabilitation practice. Goal planning in the light of teamwork and rehabilitation
- *Psychosocial effects*: Adaptation, coping. Using role-play and then applying that to the Illness Constellation Model. The professional's role in addressing individual's sexual wellbeing using the Ex-PLISSIT model
- *Evaluation of rehabilitation*: Quality of life in relation to the effectiveness of rehabilitation.

References

Heerkens Y, van der Brug Y, Ten Napel H et al 2003 Past and future use of the ICF (former IDICH) by nursing and allied health professionals. Disability and Rehabilitation 25:620–627

Jette AM, Haley SM, Kooyoomjian JT 2003 Are the ICF activity and participation dimensions distinct? Journal of Rehabilitation Medicine 35:145–149

Ogonowski JA, Kronk RA, Rice CN et al 2004 Inter-rater reliability in assigning ICF codes to children with disabilities. Disability and Rehabilitation 26:353–361

Orem D 1985 Nursing – concepts and practice, 3rd edn. Prentice-Hall, London

Parenboom RJM, Chorus AMJ 2003 Measuring participation according to the international

classification of functioning, disability and health (ICF). Disability and Rehabilitation 25:577–587

Spencer J, Hersch G, Shelton M et al 2002 Functional outcomes and daily life activities of African-American elders after hospitalisation. American Journal of Occupational Therapy 56:149–159

Wade DT, Halligan P 2003 New wine in old bottles: the WHO ICF as an explanatory model of human behaviour. Clinical Rehabilitation 17:349–354

World Health Organization 1980 The international classification of impairments, disabilities and handicaps. World Health Organization, Geneva

World Health Organization 2001 International classification of functioning, disability and health. World Health Organization, Geneva

Subject Index